Celebrate...dinner

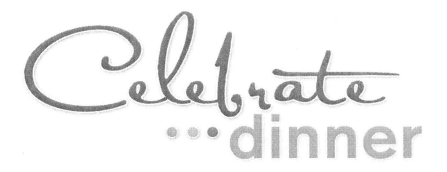

EATING GOURMET THE FRUGAL WAY!

ANITRA KERR

Bonneville Books
Springville, Utah

© 2009 Anitra Kerr

All rights reserved.

No part of this book may be reproduced in any form whatsoever, whether by graphic, visual, electronic, film, microfilm, tape recording, or any other means, without prior written permission of the publisher, except in the case of brief passages embodied in critical reviews and articles.

This is not an official publication of The Church of Jesus Christ of Latter-day Saints. The opinions and views expressed herein belong solely to the author and do not necessarily represent the opinions or views of Cedar Fort, Inc. Permission for the use of sources, graphics, and photos is also solely the responsibility of the author.

ISBN 13: 978-1-59955-306-1

Published by Bonneville Books, an imprint of Cedar Fort, Inc., 2373 W. 700 S., Springville, UT 84663
Distributed by Cedar Fort, Inc., www.cedarfort.com

LIBRARY OF CONGRESS CATALOGING-IN-PUBLICATION DATA

Kerr, Anitra, 1971–
  Celebrate dinner! : eating gourmet the food storage way / Anitra Kerr.
    p. cm.
  ISBN 978-1-59955-306-1 (acid-free paper)
 1. Cookery. 2. Menus. 3. Grocery shopping. I. Title.

TX714.K477 2009
641.5--dc22

2009017309

Cover design by Angela D. Olsen
Cover design © 2009 by Lyle Mortimer

Printed in the United States of America

10 9 8 7 6 5 4 3 2 1

Printed on acid-free paper

table of contents

A Special Thank You vi

Preface vii

Chapter 1: Put Some Zing in Your Zones 1
Chapter 2: Stocked to Please 3
Chapter 3: Refreshing the Refrigerator 7
Chapter 4: Let's Go Shopping! 9
Chapter 5: Bringing Home the Groceries 13
Chapter 6: Meal Planning with Ease 17
Chapter 7: Organizing Your Recipes 21
Chapter 8: Kid Friendly, Mother Approved 23
Chapter 9: Dealing with Picky Eaters 29
Chapter 10: Fast Food the Healthy Way 31
Chapter 11: Establish Good Habits 35
Chapter 12: Celebrate Dinner! 37

Recipes 39

A Special ••• thank you

I've always believed that a meal is just a meal until you share it with the ones you love, and then it becomes a memory! A sincere thanks to my husband and children who've helped me to realize that the simple act of gathering around the kitchen table to enjoy a meal together is always a reason to celebrate. And finally, a note of gratitude to A. Dennis Mead who has helped me edit this book, and continues to encourage me in my writing endeavors.

Preface

• • • what's for dinner?

If you've ever dreamed of hiring your own chef out of sheer frustration with the dinnertime blues, or if you feel overwhelmed at the concept of balanced meal planning, you've come to the right place. As a wife and a mother of four hungry boys, I've come to appreciate firsthand the challenges of trying to keep meal planning manageable. The shopping, the planning, the stocking, and the chopping can seem overwhelming as life just seems to get busier and busier. I know how frustrating it can be to appeal to picky eaters and to wonder if your children are getting the best nutrition possible.

Like many of you, I used to cringe at the question, "What's for dinner?" and wish I were sick and my neighbor would offer to bring in a warm meal—just for variety's sake. But those days are long gone, and I'm thrilled to share with you how I conquered those anxieties. I now not only look forward to dinnertime, but I love to shop for groceries, stock my shelves, and put on my apron every day to create simple masterpieces in the kitchen. Best of all, my family looks forward to dinner, and it's never the same thing twice in a row. We have a 91-day meal-planning schedule, and we rarely have leftovers. I shop once a week. My meals are planned by noon every day, and I am rotating my food supply regularly. I even have back-up meals in place, if I change my mind on a whim, or if I ever have to ask my husband to throw dinner together. And trust me, those meals need to be as simple as possible!

Let me show you how simple and enjoyable meal planning can be. Open your mind to the possibility of a well-stocked pantry, filled with nutritious food and matching containers. Relish the choices before you at the supermarket and bring home foods that are naturally full of color. Learn how to create healthy snacks and meals for the ones you love, and feel reenergized as you take the time to prepare foods that are full of life and nutrition. Welcome to meal planning made simple!

Chapter 1
• • • put some zing in your zones

When an artist begins to create his masterpiece, what is the first thing he does? He checks to make sure his palette is loaded and his paintbrushes are all in tip-top condition. Why? Because his tools become an extension of him as a creator, an imaginer, an artist. Similarly, we are creators in the kitchen. We have certain tools that make our job easier, and by having all the necessary supplies to create our culinary masterpieces, we can be sure that what we present to those we love is our best effort.

I like to divide my kitchen zones into four specific areas: the baking and prep zone, the cooking zone, the cleaning zone, and the "let's wrap it up" zone. As we declutter these zones and store only what is truly necessary, not only do we become more efficient in the kitchen, but our zones become clean and organized. Who needs twelve muffin pans and eight mixing bowls anyway? Be honest with yourself as you stock your zones, and try to limit yourself to three rubber spatulas and four mixing bowls. As you look through these lists, take inventory of what you have and what you'll need to make preparing everyday meals simpler and more enjoyable.

1. THE BAKING AND PREP ZONE

- variety of mixing bowls
- rubber spatulas
- baking sheets
- measuring cups and spoons
- electric mixer
- can opener
- muffin pans and loaf pans
- round and rectangle pans
- cheese grater
- vegetable peeler
- food processor
- citrus grater/juicer
- slicer/shredder
- dressing tumbler
- rolling pin
- cookie scoops

2. THE COOKING ZONE

- mandolin
- cutting board
- variety of pots and pans
- spices and herbs
- collection of knives
- ladle, pasta tool
- spatulas and wooden spoons
- wire whisks
- garlic press
- cooling racks
- trivets and pot holders
- potato masher
- sieve and colander
- kitchen shears
- fire extinguisher
- pressure cooker
- oil dispenser*

*The oil dispenser is truly essential in my kitchen. I picked up an empty ketchup bottle at my local grocery store and filled it with oil. Then I placed the bottle next to my stovetop. I use it to squirt oil into my pan when sautéing, to add oil to boiling pasta water to help keep the noodles from sticking, and even to quickly oil a baking pan. Perhaps the least expensive tool in my kitchen, it has proven to be one of my best cooking companions.

3. THE CLEANING ZONE

- variety of cleaning sprays
- trash liners
- rubber gloves
- scrubbers/brushes
- hand soap and lotion
- paper towels
- wiping cloths
- dishcloths/towels

4. THE "LET'S WRAP IT UP" ZONE

- tin foil
- plastic wrap
- storage containers
- lunch sacks
- freezer bags
- bread bags
- gallon, quart, and snack-size bags
- parchment paper
- paper and plastic ware
- bag clips/twisties

So go ahead, put some zing in your zones, and see how good it feels to have the tools you need to prepare the meals you love.

Chapter 2

stocked to please

Who doesn't love options, especially when it comes to food? Isn't it a lovely thing to open the pantry doors and be tempted by a variety of tasty foods? It's equally satisfying to look inside the refrigerator and instead of wondering if there's bread at all, being able to make a choice between sourdough, bagels, or pumpernickel. Who doesn't enjoy the peace of mind that comes from knowing the freezer is always stocked with a variety of meats, vegetables, and plenty of ice cream? A well-stocked pantry, refrigerator, and freezer space are not only convenient, but they give you the flexibility to change your dinner plans on a dime, and even entertain unexpected guests without a fuss. Here are some foods I feel are basic in maintaining these three areas:

I. IN THE PANTRY

- soup stocks
- canned fruits and veggies
- pasta sauces
- variety of pasta
- variety of beans
- rice blends*
- canned meats
- crackers and chips
- cereals
- peanut butter
- jelly, syrup, and honey
- hot cocoa
- condiments
- dried fruits and veggies
- nuts, chips
- herbs and spices
- baking items
- healthy snacks
- canned soups
- bottled juices
- pantry mixes†
- onions, potatoes

*Plain rice can get rather boring at times, so why not make up your own rice blends? Here are some simple recipes for flavored rice blends that will add some pizzazz to your everyday meal planning. Simply combine the ingredients for each rice blend, and store the mix in an airtight container on your pantry shelf.

1. Chicken Tarragon Rice Blend

4 cups uncooked long-grain rice
4 Tbsp. instant chicken bouillon
1½ tsp. sea salt
1 Tbsp. dried tarragon
1 Tbsp. dried parsley
¼ tsp. white pepper

2. Spanish Kick Rice Blend

4 cups uncooked long-grain rice
1 Tbsp. chili powder
1 Tbsp. Cumin
1½ tsp. sea salt

3. Dilly Lemon Rice Blend

4 cups uncooked long-grain rice
6 tsp. dried grated lemon peel
4 tsp. dill weed
2 tsp. dried chives
2 tsp. sea salt
3 Tbsp. instant chicken broth

4. Creamy Herb Rice Blend

4 cups uncooked long-grain rice
¼ cup dried minced celery
1 Tbsp. dried thyme
4 Tbsp. instant chicken bouillon
½ cup instant dry milk
2 Tbsp. dried parsley
1 Tbsp. dried marjoram

To prepare these rice blends, combine 2½ cups water with 1 cup rice blend and 2 Tbsp. butter in a saucepan. Bring to a boil, and then reduce the heat and simmer with the lid on until rice is tender and the water is absorbed. These blends can also be prepared by simply sautéing 1 cup rice blend with 2 tablespoons butter until golden brown, slowly adding 2½ cups water, bringing it to boil, then covering the pan, and simmering until the rice is tender and the water is all absorbed. This method of sautéing the rice first in butter is similar to packaged Rice-a-Roni found in the store, only without all the preservatives.

These flavored rice blends are delicious served as a warm side dish, or cold in a salad. I love to add fresh olives, tomatoes, basil, and chicken, and then drizzle the salad with a lovely vinaigrette. It makes a hearty meal!

†How often do you find yourself buying packaged foods like macaroni and cheese, cake mixes, and pancake mixes that are usually laden with preservatives and oftentimes even MSG? Later in this book, I'll share a few of my favorite pantry mixes made from scratch, which are, of course, preservative-free!

2. IN THE REFRIGERATOR

fresh eggs	parmesan cheese	parsley and green onions
variety of cheeses	butter	salad dressings
fresh milk	seasonal fruits	mayo and mustard
sour cream	seasonal vegetables	yogurt
variety of lunch meats	lemon	English muffins
fresh cream	breads and bagels	flour tortillas
cream cheese	garlic	

3. IN THE FREEZER

ice cream	ground beef	grated cheese
berries and fruits	stew meat	desserts
juices	pre-cooked meats	*pesto cubes
spinach and peas	pie crusts	**herb butter
chicken	vegetable mix	***chicken stock

*Although I don't claim to be an avid gardener, I do love to grow my own herbs. When I have a plentiful harvest of parsley and basil, I use them to make tantalizing pesto and herbed butter. Once the concoctions are made, I simply pour them into ice cube trays and freeze them for a few hours. Then I transfer the cubes to quart-size freezer bags or vacuum seal a dozen cubes with my food-saver vacuum sealer. Whenever I want to sauté vegetables with herbed butter or make a quick pesto sauce for pizza or pasta, I simply take the cubes that I need out of the freezer, and—just like that—I can enjoy my garden herbs all over again.

Prize-Winning Pesto

2 plump garlic cloves
1 tsp. sea salt
¼ cup toasted pine nuts
3 cups basil, loosely packed
½ cup grated parmesan cheese
¼ cup olive oil

In a food processor, blend all ingredients until smooth. Pour mixture into ice cube trays until firm. Transfer cubes to freezer bags and use when needed. Delicious for pizza topping as well as pasta sauce.

Herbed Butter

1 stick butter, softened slightly
2 Tbsp. finely chopped parsley
2 Tbsp. finely chopped basil

On a cutting board, using a wide spreader knife, gently blend all ingredients until well combined. Shape herbed butter into a log, and carefully transfer to wax paper. Wrap gently and place in the freezer. When ready to use, simply cut off 1–2 tablespoons and use to sauté vegetables, fish, or pasta.

Chicken Stock

Cooking chicken is a weekly event in my kitchen, so I like to take advantage of the moment by adding some celery, onion, and garlic to my cooking water. This way, when the chicken's done cooking, I can easily strain the broth, pour it into ice cube trays, and then store the frozen broth cubes in a bag for later use. This is what I call pure chicken broth!

Chapter 3
●●● refreshing the refrigerator

To me, having a clean refrigerator is like slipping on a pair of cool slippers after a warm bath. It's refreshing. Why not make it part of your weekly routine to tidy and wipe down the fridge before your big grocery shopping escapade? Imagine coming home to clean spaces that are waiting to be filled with fresh and nutritious foods, and knowing that you don't have to sort through leftovers to make room for it all. This simple habit of refreshing the refrigerator is just another way to help you stay organized in the kitchen. Here are some simple steps:

1. Take everything out of the fridge—yes, everything!
2. As you remove the items from the fridge, put them in groups: condiments, produce, dairy, breads, and so forth. This helps you see how much room you need when you put them all back in.
3. Wipe down the shelves and drawers.
4. With an anti-bacterial cleaning solution, clean the fridge thoroughly. I like to take fresh paper towels and line my produce and meat drawers with them, just in case I have leaks; then my drawers don't get sticky.
5. Look at all the food you pulled out and ask yourself what can be thrown away and what goes back into the fridge. If you have leftovers, put them back close to the front so you can give them first priority. Wipe down bottles if necessary.
6. Each food has a home. Organize your food, just as you would your pantry. Grouping foods helps you save time when you're in a hurry. Here are my tips:

a. Dairy products on the top shelf—eggs, yogurt, sour cream, cottage cheese
b. Breads on the second shelf—bagels, tortillas, English muffins
c. "Now" foods on the next shelf—leftovers, perishables, desserts
d. Meats and cheeses in their own drawers
e. Produce in their own drawers
f. Milks, juices, condiments, dressings in the fridge doors

By organizing and cleaning your fridge before the shopping trip, you'll know exactly what you have, and you'll make room for what's about to come. This is an important step in keeping foods fresh and helping maintain order in your meal-planning.

Chapter 4
let's go shopping!

Hooray! Let's go shopping! Who says grocery shopping has to be boring? How many of us feel like the grocery store is our second home? Well, it certainly doesn't have to be. Wouldn't it be nice to frequent the grocery store only once a week instead of every night right before dinner? Can you imagine the time you'd save during the week by simply "picking up" your groceries at home from your own "grocery shelves" instead of combing the aisles every afternoon at the downtown supermarket? I suggest you choose a particular day and a particular time each week that you do your grocery shopping, and then get it all done in one trip. That's right—one trip. If you're like me, you'll shop at one warehouse-type establishment, where you can purchase items in bulk. You may also have a favorite neighborhood grocery store where you pick up your fresh produce and specialty items. Regardless of where you shop, there is one important thing to always take with you. And I'm not talking about the cash—I'm talking about the shopping list. If there's one thing that will help keep you focused on the sometimes daunting task at hand, it's that very specific grocery list. By creating a master grocery list, you can quickly move through the store, picking up the items you need, and avoid being tempted by the things you don't. Remember once you've created this master grocery list, you'll never have to make one again. You'll simply add to it week by week as you see fit. Here are the steps:

1. Begin with a pen and paper.
2. You may want to invite someone to help you write, as you dictate, because your list may be quite long.

3. Make your list.
4. Continue, as if aisle by aisle, and jot down your staple foods—those you'd buy the most often.
5. Divide the items into categories.
6. When you come home from the store, divide those items into sections, or by aisle, whichever is easiest for you. For example: produce, canned goods, cleaning products, and so forth (see example on the next page).
7. Create a master list.
8. After categorizing your items, make a master list on your computer. Save the file because you will occasionally add to it. You may want to make the font small enough to fit two or three copies on one page. Make 52 copies of this master list—one for each week of the year. Place these copies somewhere you'll remember.
9. Post your list.

Every week, you'll post this master list either on your fridge or bulletin board. Instead of writing down every last item you need, all you need to do is circle the items on the list that you need that week. Simple as that! If you need to add to it, write it in. Be sure to let your family know they can add to this list as well. Take it to the store with you, and stick to it! When you've finished shopping, throw that list away, and immediately post a new master list for the coming week.

MASTER GROCERY LIST

PAPER GOODS	CLEANING SUPPLIES	PERSONAL HYGIENE
towels	toilet/floor	razors/deodorants
toilet paper	countertop cleaner	feminine products
foil/Saran wrap	stainless steel	toothpaste/floss
garbage bags	Windex	bath soap/bubbles
napkins/plates/cups	laundry/dish soap	shampoo/conditioner
plastic utensils	fabric softener	tips/cotton balls
Ziploc bags/lunch sacks	furniture polish	

let's go shopping! • 11

DAIRY PRODUCTS
milk/butter
yogurt/sour cream
whipped cream
cottage cheese
parmesan cheese
cream cheese
assorted cheeses
eggs

DELI
specialty breads
cheeses
meats
bagels
spreads

EVERY DAY
chips
cereals
hot cocoa/drinks
peanut butter/jelly
honey/syrup
salsa
pasta sauce
rice
pasta
canned goods

FROZEN FOODS
ice cream
fruits/vegetables
desserts
chicken
shrimp
meatballs
juice

CONDIMENTS
ketchup/mustard
mayo/Dijon
olives
dressing
soy sauce
broths

OTHER

PRODUCE
lettuce/spinach
celery/carrots
lemons/limes
green onions/parsley
onions/garlic
apples/bananas
melons
berries

BAKING SUPPLIES
flour/sugar
spices/chips
nuts/dried fruits
cocoa/oil

OTHER

Chapter 5
bringing home the groceries

Once you've cleaned out the refrigerator and done your grocery shopping, you're now ready to bring those groceries home. Try to allow yourself time when you come home to unwrap and rearrange your food so it can be prepared quickly and easily later. First, remove the produce items from their original bags and trim them, discarding extra leaves, bulk roots—such as those found on celery—and other extra tag-alongs like onion skins, twist ties, or grapes that may be bruised. Replace the original store bags with your choice of better quality zipper bags or plastic containers. I like using good quality bread bags for my large produce like spinach and lettuce. Then I like to protect my more delicate produce-like parsley, green onions, berries, and avocados in click-lid plastic containers. Other smaller items such as lemons, cucumbers, or tomatoes simply go in an "extras" open container in my produce drawer. This way, I'm assured those smaller items aren't buried underneath a big bag of carrots or a bundle of lettuce. This extra little container is also ideal to pull out when making salads and sandwiches, because all the items are together. Wipe off the fruits, place grapes in a bowl, and even chop some of your fresh vegetables for quick snacks. These make a great alternative to sugary munchies.

Second, let's discuss how to store meats. If you purchase your meat in bulk—for example, chicken breasts, ground beef, fish, or stew meat—consider dividing up those items into meal-size portions. I like to use a vacuum sealer to store foods such as this in the freezer. This way I can avoid freezer burn and save space in the freezer as well. You may want to go one step further and pre-cook some of these meats. For example, if you buy a ten-pound package of ground beef, consider browning five pounds of that beef along with some onions and a little garlic, and then freezing that meat in one-pound portions. When pre-cooking chicken breasts, perhaps you could add a little celery, onions, and salt to the cooking water, and when the chicken is cooked, simply cube the chicken and freeze and strain the vegetables from the broth. Pour the clear broth into ice-cube trays and set the trays in the freezer, later transferring those broth cubes to a separate freezer bag. This way, next time you need chicken broth, simply pull out your broth cubes and you've got a head start on a delicious soup! When purchasing lunch meats, it's a good idea to group them with sliced cheeses in a "sandwich making kit" in your refrigerator. This kit is nothing more than a container to hold all your sandwich items together. This makes creating tasty sandwiches a cinch.

Third, let's talk about cheese. I find it much more economical to purchase cheese in bulk, rather than buying it in one-pound blocks or having it sliced at the deli. I look for the largest cheese loaf I can find, then divide the cheese myself when I come home. I use a food processor with different blades—one that quickly slices the cheese and another that grates the cheese. This gives me options without spending extra money on packaging. Once I slice the cheese, I put it into uniform stacks and wrap it tightly in cellophane. This will go into my "sandwich making kit" mentioned earlier. Any specialty cheeses are purchased in small quantities and can also fit in this kit.

Fourth on our list is cereal. Have you ever stopped to count how many boxes of cereal are on your shelf? Of all those boxes, how many are the same? Do you find yourself buying more cereal before the last box is gone just because you're just not quite sure how much is left, but you don't want to have to open each box to find out? Well let me give you a simpler solution. If you're like most people, you buy the same cereals over and over again. We all have our favorites. Why not get rid of the boxes once and for all and just start storing your cereals in clear plastic food-grade containers? This way, you always know how much you have; the container is labeled, in case you forget what you had when you run out. Best of all, you're eliminating clutter and multiple packages in your pantry. And it gets even better—did you know the average cereal box is close to one gallon in bulk? Is it any surprise, then, that manufacturers sell their food-grade containers in one-gallon sizes? There's your perfect match! As you learn to transfer foods from their original containers into clear containers, not only does it eliminate the guesswork, but it gives your pantry the appearance and the feel of order and cleanliness.

Now on to our last group of foods: baking supplies. When arriving home from the grocery store, it may be tempting to throw those bags of chocolate chips, coconut, marshmallows, or flour right in the pantry in their original bags. But what happens when those bags get opened for the first time? Are you going to cinch them up with a rubber band, or fold the bag over, hoping it won't open and spill, or gently squeeze it into the corner of the cupboard and forget about it all together? Certainly not! As we discussed earlier, the more efficient way to keep these foods fresh and handy is to place them in individual containers with screw-top lids. They'll stack easily, and best of all, your cupboards will stay clean and clutter-free.

One of the greatest challenges to storing food is creating a system whereby the food can be organized efficiently. Whether you have a large walk-in pantry or simply a few kitchen cupboards, learning to keep similar foods together by containerizing them can help meal planning and general food preparation be simple and easy. Not only does proper containerizing help maximize your storage space, but your pantry and cupboards will stay cleaner longer, and you and your family members will be more likely to find what you're looking for without having to dig through half-empty bags and open packages. When similar items are packaged the same way, there is a natural sense of order and cleanliness. Who doesn't appreciate that in the kitchen? When working with clients in home organization, one of the challenges I regularly face is helping people understand how to choose the best container for each food group in their pantry. Let me share a few ideas with you.

1. **Cereals:** 1-gallon clear plastic screw-top containers
2. **Pastas and beans:** 1-gallon and ½-gallon clear plastic screw-top containers
3. **Baking supplies** (baking chips, coconut, sugars, marshmallows): ½-gallon clear plastic screw-top containers
4. **Nuts and dried fruit:** ¼-gallon clear plastic screw-top containers
5. **Herbs and spices:** 3-6-oz. glass screw-top jars with wide-mouth lids

Of course, a container just wouldn't be as impressive without a label affixed to the front, so keep your labeler close at hand, and label, label, label.

Chapter 6
meal planning with ease

So much of successful meal preparation is really in the planning. If you can become comfortable with the shopping, the stocking, and the scheduling, you're 99 percent of the way there. Now comes the fun part—creating a meal planning calendar. Do you ever get tired of the same meal routine, eating the same ten meals over and over again? Well, let me introduce you to a refreshing way to make everything in your pantry count. This is a great way to prepare a wide variety of meals, while wisely rotating your food supply. Here we go.

1. LOOK AT YOUR PANTRY

You may have ten different items, or you may have a hundred. Each of these foods will become an ingredient in your dinner menus. Let's take a can of olives, for example. Think of three meals you can make with olives: Navajo tacos, chicken enchiladas, and barbecue pizzas. That's easy; let's try another. How about tomato sauce? I'm thinking of minestrone, homemade pasta sauce, and stuffed cabbage rolls. Do you see how simple this exercise is? I challenge you to come up with three dinner menus you can use with each item in your pantry. This is the beginning to creating your own list of dinner menus. If you don't have recipes, visit the library, ask a friend to share their favorites, or simply Google the ingredient for tasty ways to use each of those foods you have stored. Don't be afraid to expand your culinary horizons.

2. CREATE A "FAMILY'S FAVORITES" LIST

You may have ten or twenty favorite meals. The ingredients for those dishes should take first priority when stocking your pantry. Make sure you have enough ingredients to prepare those meals eight to ten times. Important: Consider how you would substitute the fresh ingredients in each recipe with canned, dehydrated, or freeze-dried varieties. After all, these are your favorite meals, and comfort is key. You never know when those fresh ingredients may be temporarily unavailable, and it's always a good idea to have a back-up plan.

3. PLAN WELL-BALANCED MEALS

By incorporating a wide variety of foods into our daily diets, we not only feel better, but our families will actually look forward to dinnertime. Shake it up! Instead of getting stuck eating chicken dishes over and over, or resorting to spaghetti too often, why not divide your week into theme days?

THE MEAL PLANNING CALENDAR

The most helpful way I have found to plan dinners for my family is to create a meal planning calendar. All you need is a wall calendar, with boxes that are 1½ inches square. You'll want to purchase some narrow colored sticky tabs to write your dinner entrees on. These will be removed every so often and transferred from one month to another, depending on how many times you choose to repeat those meals. Here's how the meal planning calendar works:

1. Write down your favorite meals
2. Whether you start with 10 meals or 90 meals, it's the same concept. You can always add more sticky tabs as your list grows. Use one sticky tab for each dinner idea. I like to color-code mine for convenience:
   Blue: soup
   Purple: salad and bread
   Yellow: pasta
   Pink: beef
   Orange: chicken
   Green: beans or vegetarian
3. Try to alternate colors so you're not repeating the same item over and over.

LEARN TO CREATE YOUR SHOPPING LIST QUICKLY

Now that you have your master shopping list and your menu ideas, finalizing that list should be a cinch. Simply circle the items you'll need to supplement for the menus you've planned, and be sure to review the master list to see if you're low on any other items. Making a habit of purchasing multiple items can help you avoid unnecessary shopping trips. For example, if you need a bottle of ketchup, consider buying three more while you're at it, because chances are if you need it once, you'll need it again. And what usually happens when we go to the store for just one thing? We usually come out with ten more different items.

TIP: When you're planning your menus, try to serve sooner those foods that need to be eaten in the beginning of the week, for example fresh strawberries, green onions, and others. If you think some of those items won't be eaten all in one dinner, plan to prepare another dinner using those same ingredients.

Example: I like to make an Asian chicken salad that calls for green onions. I don't need the whole bunch for one meal, so I'll plan to make my chicken salad on Monday, and then serve beef enchiladas on Thursday, and sprinkle the green onions on top of those. Those green onions will not go to waste!

ESTABLISH A REGULAR TIME FOR DINNER PREPARATIONS

If you can, try to have dinner preparations done by 11 AM. This frees up the rest of your day, and you won't feel the dinnertime crunch at 4 PM. If you plan to serve rolls, start the dough in the morning. If your vegetables need to be chopped, do them early. If you're preparing a casserole, prepare it in the morning, and wrap it stored in the fridge so it's ready to pop into the oven right before dinner.

HONESTLY EVALUATE DINNER

A big part of successful menu planning is to decide if the meals you prepare are worth repeating. If your dinner was a success, take the sticky tab off that calendar date and place it on a later calendar date, to be repeated. If the dinner you made wasn't a real hit, don't worry! Just grab another sticky tab, and choose another dinner entrée using the same basic theme we discussed above. I have been guilty of taking rejection of my dinners personally, and felt like crawling into fetal position on my bed. It's ridiculous, and embarrassing to admit, but it happens to all of us, right? Instead, let's just deal with such events and count them as valuable learning experiences. Because I love to have 91 different meals to choose from, I know three months in advance what I'll be serving for dinner. You can too!

BE FLEXIBLE

Dinnertime is not an exact science, as we all know. Allow yourself a blank sticky tab once in a while. Consider serving breakfast foods for dinner, have leftovers, or eat out. I don't always stick to my dinner menus if I find that my mood screams for something different!

Chapter 7
organizing your recipes

Do you have more recipe books than you know what to do with? Do you ever feel frustrated because you can't remember which cookbook has which recipes? Let me give you a few ideas to help you sift through the clutter.

Browse through all your cookbooks. Place a sticky tab on all the ones you want to keep. If you have a whole cookbook but only use two or three recipes, consider cutting out those recipes along with the pictures and placing them in a large binder with plastic pages. Then cheerfully donate the original recipe book to your local recycling center. If you have loose recipes in a box, consider retyping them and saving them to a file. As you add to the file, simply print the recipes on index cards and place them in your large recipe binder. Divide the recipes with tabs: dinners, desserts, soups, salads, and so forth. For quick references to frequently used recipes, consider taping those index cards to the inside of an upper kitchen cabinet near your work zone. Then all you have to do is open the cupboard, prepare the recipes, and close the cupboard again. It's that easy! I especially like to use this method for breads, pancakes, and cookies. It also makes it easy for my children to find the recipes we make most often.

If you want to separate your food storage recipes into a special binder, divide those recipes into sections like beans, powdered dairy, grains, dehydrated foods, and so forth. I have found that my food storage is just an extension of my pantry, and because I'm always rotating my items equally, I like all my recipes to be stored together, food storage, or not. Keep only those cookbooks that you can't part with. Donate the rest to charity, or use the pictures to decorate your recipe binder.

If you have young children or grandchildren, you may enjoy helping them put together a collection of their favorite recipes as well, teaching them how to make simple meals or snacks in the kitchen. This encourages independence and an appreciation for good food and healthy habits.

Chapter 8

kid friendly, mother approved

I have always believed that the relationship between a mother and a child is enhanced when great food is prepared and shared in the home kitchen. I also believe that once we teach our children independence in the kitchen, it helps to develop within them self-confidence in making healthy choices. So, speaking of independence, why not start by teaching our children to prepare their own lunches for school? By making the foods easily accessible, and by providing healthy choices, children can enjoy taking part in this daily routine. Here are some things to have on hand:

- lunch sacks and plastic baggies (these should be stored low where children can easily reach them)
- prepared snack bags to grab and go
- sliced bread
- variety of cheeses and meats for sandwiches
- washed and torn lettuce
- easy-squeeze mayo and mustard
- peanut butter and jelly
- plastic knives to spread items on bread
- cleaned fruits
- chopped vegetables or baby carrots
- healthy desserts, like trail mix, fruit cups, etc.
- canned drinks or bottled water
- string cheese
- mini bags of popped corn
- crackers or mini muffins
- baked chips

MORE ABOUT SNACKS

After-school snack time can also be a challenge for some, because many kids go for the sugary snacks. But with a little planning, you too can offer your children a healthier alternative. I like to have a snack basket in the pantry, stocked with items like oatmeal packets, granola bars, baked crackers, popcorn, dried fruits, and fruit leather. I also have a section in the fridge dedicated to after-school snacks. This section has yogurt, string cheese, fruit, cut-up vegetables, and so forth. Our rule is: only two after-school snacks per child. It's a good idea to have snack items pre-measured so that kids don't overeat. Too many snacks, and their dinner appetites are gone! Let them choose which two they prefer, but snack time ends at 4:00.

Below are some delicious recipes for after-school snacking, whether it's you or the kiddies who indulge in them!

HEALTHY SNACKS FOR HAPPY KIDS

Frozen Yogurt Pineapple Pops

2 cups vanilla yogurt
1 can crushed pineapple
mini cups
tin foil
wooden popsicle sticks

In a blender, combine the yogurt and undrained pineapple. Blend well, and then pour into mini cups, about $2/3$ full. Cover each cup with a square of tin foil; then slit the foil with a knife. Insert the wooden stick, and then transfer cups to the freezer until solid (about 2 hours). Gently pull out the yogurt pops, and enjoy!

Disappearing Zucchini Mini Muffins

1½ cups shredded zucchini
2 cups biscuit mix
1 tsp. cinnamon
1 tsp. allspice

2 eggs
¾ cups brown sugar
½ cup applesauce
2 tsp. lemon juice
powdered sugar

Squeeze the shredded zucchini in a paper towel to get all the water out. In a bowl, combine the biscuit mix, cinnamon, and allspice. In a separate bowl, mix the eggs, brown sugar, applesauce, and lemon juice. Combine both mixtures until smooth, and then spoon into paper-lined mini muffin cups. Bake at 375 degrees for 10–15 minutes or until muffins are done. When cooled, sprinkle with powdered sugar.

Incredible Edible Veggie Bowl

1 red, yellow, or orange pepper, washed and seeded
celery sticks
carrot sticks
salad dressing

With a knife, cut the pepper in half, discarding the seeds and paring the ribs. Use half of the pepper as the serving bowl, and slice the other half into thin strips. Place a little salad dressing in the bottom of the pepper bowl, and then fill the bowl with carrot, pepper, and celery sticks. When the veggies are gone, you can eat the bowl as well.

Peanut Butter Apple Disks

2 apples
4 Tbsp. peanut butter
2 Tbsp. granola

Wash, core, and slice the apples. Spread peanut butter on the disks, and then sprinkle with granola.

Frozen Grape Jewels

Take a bunch of red grapes and freeze them individually in a Ziploc bag. When you want a refreshing snack, grab the grapes and pop them into your mouth. This is also a great way to add some sparkle to your dinner water. It keeps the water cold, and your family enjoys the treat.

Granola Bars

½ cup crunchy peanut butter
½ cup corn syrup
½ cup brown sugar
1 tsp. vanilla
3 cups prepared granola

In a small saucepan, melt the peanut butter, corn syrup, brown sugar, and vanilla. Pour over the prepared granola. Mix until well blended. Press the granola mixture into a shallow baking pan. Allow to cool. Cut into bars, and sprinkle with chocolate chips if desired. Package each bar in parchment paper, and secure with tape.

Classic Trail Mix

4 cups Chex Mix
½ cup dried fruit
½ cup craisins or raisins
½ cup peanuts
½ cup M&Ms
¼ cup pumpkin seeds, optional

Combine all ingredients and store in individual snack-size bags.

Apple Cinnamon Fruit Roll-ups

²/₃ blender full of cinnamon applesauce
½ cup water

Combine all ingredients in a blender until smooth. Pour onto lightly greased fruit leather trays. Makes 3 trays. Dry 10 hours or until dry. Roll up leather, wrap in plastic, and then cut into 2-inch sections. Perfect for lunches or after-school snacks.

Instant Oatmeal Packets

In each snack-size bag, place the following:

¼ cup rolled oats
2 Tbsp. ground rolled oats
2 Tbsp. powdered milk
pinch of sea salt
1 Tbsp. brown sugar
½ tsp. cinnamon

When ready to eat, simply add ¾ cups milk or water to a bowl, dump in the oatmeal packet, and microwave for 90 seconds. (Optional additions: raisins, nutmeg, dried apple flakes, etc.)

Popped Wheaties

Popped wheat is crunchy like a chip but so much more healthy. You can season it with anything you like.

2 Tbsp. oil
½ cup cooked wheat berries
seasonings of your choice

In a frying pan, heat oil until little bubbles appear. Carefully add the cooked wheat, and spread it thinly in the pan. Cover with a lid, and allow to cook over medium heat until you hear popping and the wheat turns golden brown. Be careful not to burn the wheat.

Transfer onto a paper towel to allow oil to drain, and pat a little. Then season with any seasoning you'd like. (Barbecue or cinnamon sugar are my family's favorites.) Cool completely. Store in a container in the pantry.

Chapter 9
dealing with picky eaters

Many of us are "blessed" with picky eaters. So what do we do to reduce the tears at mealtime while making sure our children get the nutrition they need? I have dealt with this issue for years and have found some simple solutions. I always wanted to believe in the statement, "When they're hungry, they'll eat anything!" But that has simply never worked in my home. Some children would rather go to bed than eat dinner with the family, and that doesn't solve any problems. In fact, it can create feelings of anxiety and cause contention and embarrassment with family members, especially Mom!

I believe mealtime should be a happy time. Each member of the family should look forward to dinner and not cower in fear of what's coming. Often, small adjustments can make a huge difference. There's no need to make one dinner for the picky eaters and make another for the others. I find that by using the same basic ingredients, I can make one meal idea into two, simply by changing the combination or the presentation. This seems to please everyone. Let me give you an example:

NORMAL	PICKY EATERS
Meal One	
Italian chicken with rice	chicken fingers, rice
shredded carrot and pineapple salad	carrot sticks, and apple slices

Meal Two	
ham and swiss paninis	grilled cheese sandwiches
spinach and carrot bisque	spinach and shredded carrots
Meal Three	
salisbury steak	hamburgers
mashed potatoes	homemade french fries

In these three meals, you'll notice I used identical ingredients but just presented them a little differently. This allows picky eaters to feel included, while being exposed to a more grown-up way to eat simple foods. Give it a try. It works!

Chapter 10

● ● ● fast food the healthy way

How many times do you find yourself at a loss half an hour before dinnertime, wondering what to make with what you have? Do you find yourself running to the grocery store, combing up and down the aisles, and praying something will jump out at you to save the night? We all have fallen prey to busy days and hectic schedules, but I still believe there are solutions to dinner crunch times. Let me share two simple concepts with you.

I. THE PRESSURE COOKER

Many of us cringe at the words *pressure cooker*. We may have memories of food exploding on the stovetop or may be annoyed at that whistle that beckons us to beware of danger ahead. But those are days of the past! Let me introduce you to a whole new breakthrough in pressure cooking. I recently discovered one of my favorite kitchen companions in the Nesco Electric 3-in-1 pressure cooker. It's a digital pressure cooker that sits right on your countertop and is simple to operate. Not only that, but it looks great with a lovely stainless steel finish and a sleek black lid. This five-quart pressure cooker is my answer to fast food. It not only works as a pressure cooker, but also as a slow cooker and a steamer. That's right! Wave good-bye to your cumbersome Crock-Pot, your ugly rice cooker, and your bulky vegetable steamer. This 3-in-1 pressure cooker will replace them all. One of the most convenient features of this pressure cooker is the delay timer, which allows me to set a timer, leave the house, and come home to a finished meal at the touch of a button. Another great feature is a browning feature. This allows me to brown my meats and sauté my vegetables in the same pot, then add in the rest of the ingredients to finish off my masterpiece. You can't do that in a Crock-Pot!

Many of the recipes you'll find in this book can be prepared in this pressure cooker. Try out your digital pressure cooker with my tasty chili recipe, found in chapter 12. I use my pressure cooker at least three to four times a week. One of the things I never tire of is taking frozen chicken, adding ½ cup of water to the pressure cooker, and turning on my machine for 15 minutes. After the cooker comes to pressure, the digital clock starts counting down, and in just 15 minutes, my chicken is tender and falling apart—no mess, no foam, no fuss. Another food I love to cook in my pressure cooker is beans. I don't enjoy cooking beans on the stovetop. Besides taking so long, I find the smell offensive, and it's messy. Instead, I now soak my beans overnight just like I would normally, but then put them into the pressure cooker, and in 35 minutes my beans are cooked to perfection—no mess, no smell, and best of all, not mushy. I enjoy the convenience of pushing a button, walking away, and letting the pressure cooker do all the work. When the food's done cooking, I take the removable cooking bowl out of the pressure cooker, and the cleanup's a cinch.

Among all these great features of the pressure cooker, perhaps the most important of all is the nutritional benefit. Did you know that cooking foods at high pressure for a shorter amount of time helps retain much more of your food's nutritional value, like vitamins and minerals? Can you imagine steaming broccoli for two minutes instead of fifteen? How about cooking potatoes in eight minutes instead of twenty-five? Best of all, your vegetables don't become mushy, as they would when using a Crock-Pot. They're deliciously cooked to perfection, and you can feel good knowing you're preparing foods that will offer your family the best nutrition. Here's another bonus: you can even prepare desserts in your pressure cooker. The possibilities are endless, and I guarantee you, once you start using a pressure cooker, you'll have your own built-in fast food solution!

2. DINNER IN A BAG

This concept is brilliant, and I can say that, because it's not my own. The "Dinner in a Bag" idea comes from a great lady named Christine Van Wagenen, who has compiled a book of quick back-up dinner ideas, using ingredients found both in your food storage and in your fridge. By assembling what you can ahead of time, such as canned and dried goods, and then simply adding from your fridge what you need to supplement each recipe, you can have back-up meal plans ready to go. Let me explain.

One of my favorite recipes from Christine's book, *Dinner in a Bag*, is Hawaiian Luau. The recipe begins by describing all the ingredients I need to place in my bag. I like to use heavy paper bags with jute handles. You can find these at any party supply store or even in some grocery stores.

1 (10-oz.) can of cream of chicken soup
1 (10-oz.) can mandarin oranges
1 (20-oz.) can pineapple tidbits
1 cup shredded coconut (in a Ziploc bag)
1 cup cashews or almonds (in a Ziploc bag)
2 cups uncooked white rice (in a Ziploc bag)
1 cup Chinese noodles (in a container)
2 (10-oz.) cans chicken

I arrange all of these ingredients in my paper bag, and then I slip the recipe card in a plastic sleeve and add the recipe to the bag. When I'm ready to make the meal, I simply refer to the recipe card that tells me the fresh ingredients I need to have ready, as well as how to put the recipe together. Here are the ingredients I'll need to add fresh:

2 cups grated cheese
1 cup grated carrots
3 Tbsp. chopped green onions
1 cup diced tomatoes
4 cups water
salt to taste

Then I look at the directions to put all of these ingredients together:

Combine rice with 4 cups water and 1 teaspoon salt in a pot and bring to a boil. Cover and reduce heat to low, and let it simmer for 20 minutes. Remove rice from heat source and let stand covered for 10 minutes, then fluff with a fork. Warm soup, adding enough milk to make it the consistency of gravy. Add a couple dashes of soy sauce or curry powder for added flavor. Drain the fruits. Place the fruits, nuts, noodles, coconut, chicken, and desired additional ingredients in individual serving bowls. Arrange on a plate in the following order: Chinese noodles, warm rice, warm cooked chicken, vegetables, gravy, cheese, pineapple, oranges, coconut, and nuts.

Doesn't this sound delicious? And to think Christine's already done most of the work for you! In her book, *Dinner in a Bag*, she has over 40 dinner recipes that you can choose from. Each has a variety of canned and dry goods, fresh ingredients, and of course, the directions on how to create those delicious meals. Not only are these a great "fast food" idea, but they make great neighbor gifts. Think of a new mom who'd love to have three or four meals ready to put together at her own leisure, or an elderly neighbor who could use help once in a while with a decorated "Dinner in a Bag." Encourage your children to help you put some of these bags together and teach them the value of planning ahead and creating simple meals from the pantry.

To purchase your copy of Christine's *Dinner in a Bag*, contact:

Help U Mail
10291 South 1300 East
Sandy, Utah 84094
(801) 571-1441

So, look forward to your back-up plan. Don't be caught in the grocery aisles at ten minutes to six wondering what to make for dinner anymore. Learn the value of a pressure cooker, prepare some back-up dinner meals, and let "busyness" happen elsewhere!

Chapter 11
establish good habits

Learning to implement concepts of efficient meal planning takes time, so be patient with yourself, and have fun. Involve your family members in selecting dinner menus, in meal-time preparations, and in the cleanup. Setting a daily or weekly routine will help meal planning run more smoothly. Here are just a few suggestions:

- Establish a regular meal time, and stick to it.
- Set aside a regular shopping day and time, and don't linger.
- Create and stick to a master grocery list.
- Clean your refrigerator before grocery shopping.
- Learn to delegate responsibilities among family members. This could include setting the table, emptying the trash, unloading the dishwasher, and so forth.
- Put together some back-up meals as discussed in chapter 10 and consider that as your "fast food" option.
- Have clean dish cloths, towels, and fresh trash liners in your kitchen every morning.

Make sure the dishes get done before bed so you can start fresh every day. As you begin to implement the concepts I've discussed in this book, remember to take baby steps. Begin by organizing your kitchen space, arranging your tools, and stocking up on those time-saving accessories that will help your meal preparation go faster and run more smoothly. Next, move on to your pantry space, making order and efficiency your top priority. Group your foods in similar groups, making them easier to access. Choose containers that allow you to see your food and know when it's time to restock. Promise yourself to learn how to use each food that you store, and make it a habit to rotate through all your foods regularly through sensible meal planning. Take a look at your refrigerator and freezer space, and schedule regular cleanings to make sure these spaces are well stocked but not over-loaded.

Allow yourself time to take care of your foods upon return from the grocery store, replacing cheap bags, dividing large quantities of foods into meal-size portions, and making sure fruits and vegetables are always front and center upon opening the fridge. This will entice those who open the fridge to make healthier choices more often. Learn to be consistent with your grocery list. Use it, stick to it, and encourage other family members to use it as well, so that you're not running to the grocery store several times a week and trying to cater to everyone's whims. Take the time to plan healthy and nutritious meals.

In the next chapter, I'll help you create a variety of delicious dinner entrees using whole grains, fresh fruits and vegetables, lean meats, and delectable herbs. As you plan and serve a healthy variety of foods, you'll find that you and your family will actually look forward to dinner at home, and dinnertime will become an event that is cherished, not a necessity that is feared.

Learn to be flexible with your plans. Be content to serve breakfast for dinner on occasion, or simply to enjoy a salad from the garden. Many of us have children or grandchildren. Let's teach them the value of independence in the kitchen by encouraging them to help us prepare foods, stock pantry shelves, and discuss healthy alternatives. Teach them to put together their own lunches once they're capable, and let's make snack time an opportunity to nourish them with whole grains, real fruit, and foods that not only build muscle, but a healthy brain! Let's not get caught in the "picky eater" trap and assume that kids will never change. Instead, consider simplifying their foods and including them in meal time planning so they can learn to make healthy choices, no matter where they go. Appreciate the abundance of beautiful food that's available in each season, and enjoy the uniqueness of new-found foods—a creamy aged cheese, a fresh catch of fish, a crusty herbed bread. Love food—the planning, the storing, the learning, the sharing. Learn to celebrate dinner!

Chapter 12
••• celebrate dinner!

I love food! I love to prepare it and experiment with it, and I love to watch the satisfaction of those who sit down to enjoy it with me. Dinnertime should be celebrated. It's a time of gathering, a time to enjoy a healthy meal with the ones you love and to share the events of the day. Unfortunately, many of us get caught in the "dinner trap." We find ourselves serving the same 10 meals over and over again, because we know those recipes by heart, and we simply don't have the time to expand our culinary horizons. Let me help you expand those horizons. I've put together my favorite 91 dinner entrées, filled with healthy, fresh, and delicious dinner ideas. Of course, since there are 91, you'll only be making each entrée 4 times during the whole year, not 36 times. Now, that should get you excited! And I've added another bonus—24 kid-friendly recipes that show you how to adapt virtually any meal into simpler creations, using the same ingredients you'd use for the rest of the family. I've also included several dinner recipes that can be made using the electric pressure cooker.

Many of the ingredients used to make these dinner recipes come straight from my food storage, like dry beans, powdered dairy products, and freeze-dried vegetables. But most of the ingredients are fresh. I find that by incorporating a lot of fresh produce with many of my pantry items, I can achieve a good balance when planning meals. It feels good to know that I have a back-up plan when certain fruits and vegetables are either not in season or not available. That's where my freeze-dried fruits and vegetables come in handy. I use them regularly in soups and other baked creations. I feel as comfortable using freeze-dried and dehydrated foods and powders as I do fresh, because I make it a habit to incorporate them into my everyday meal planning. Hopefully by experimenting with these recipes, you too will find how simple it is to treat your food storage as just an extension of your pantry, rather than as a "store and ignore" warehouse.

Whether you choose to select your favorite recipes, or decide to make these entrées part of your everyday meal planning, you'll love the variety, and your family will look forward to dinner every night!

Remember, nothing says "I love you" like a great meal can. So let's celebrate dinner!

BREADS/ SOUPS

Pumpkin Waffles with Apple Cider Syrup 40
Multi-grain Crackers 42
Meatball Minestrone with Cornbread 43
Chicken Tortilla Soup 45
Vegetable Minestrone 46
Clam Chowder 47
Taco Soup 48
Chunky Bacon Potato Soup 49
Broccoli Cheese Soup in Bread Bowls 51
French Onion Soup 52
Red Bean and Beef Borsht 53
Pasta and Chickpea Soup 54
Herbed Corn Chowder 55
Cauliflower and Blue Cheese Soup 56
Cheese Tortellini Soup 57
Chicken Noodle and Quinoa Soup 58
Autumn Harvest Split Pea Soup 59
Garden Vegetable Tabouleh Stew 60
Navy Bean and Bacon Chowder 61
Ravioli and Cabbage Soup 62

pumpkin waffles with *Apple Cider Syrup*

Every once in a while, I love to serve breakfast for dinner. These waffles are simply delicious, and they're a great companion to hash brown potatoes for a hearty meal.

Waffles

2 ½ cups flour
4 tsp. baking powder
2 tsp. cinnamon
1 tsp. allspice
1 tsp. ground ginger
½ tsp. salt
¼ cup packed brown sugar
1 cup canned pumpkin

2 cups milk
4 eggs, separated
¼ cup melted butter

Combine all dry ingredients in a mixing bowl. In another bowl, stir the liquid ingredients and the egg yolks together. Whip the egg whites in a separate bowl until stiff. Stir flour mixture and ¼ cup melted butter into the pumpkin mixture, stirring to combine. Fold in egg whites. Pour into waffle iron, and serve with hot Apple Cider Syrup (see following page for recipe).

Apple Cider Syrup

½ cup white sugar
1 Tbsp. cornstarch
1 tsp. cinnamon
1 cup apple cider
1 Tbsp. lemon juice
2 Tbsp. butter

Stir together all dry ingredients. Stir in cider and lemon juice. Cook in a small saucepan until the mixture boils and thickens. Add the butter; then remove the syrup from the heat. Serve over warm waffles.

multi-grain crackers

Preheat oven to 300 degrees. Then grind 1/3 cup of each of the following grains in your electric grinder:

kamut
quinoa
sweet brown rice
oat groats

Add the following ingredients to your flour in a large mixing bowl:

¾ cups white flour
2 Tbsp. rolled oats
¼ cup butter, sliced
1 cup water plus 3 Tbsp. butter milk powder
1½ tsp. salt
seasoning of your choice
½ tsp. baking soda

Knead until the dough is soft, about 3 minutes. Roll out dough on a countertop. Then transfer dough onto the back of a cookie sheet by draping it over your rolling pin first. Using a pizza cutter, score the dough into diamond or square shapes, and bake until slightly golden (10 minutes). Transfer crackers to a plate, and watch them disappear!

meatball minestrone
and Cornbread

1 (12 to 16-oz.) pkg. frozen cooked meatballs
3 (14-oz.) cans beef broth
1 can Great Northern Beans, rinsed and drained
1 (14 oz.) can diced stewed tomatoes
1 (10-oz.) pkg. frozen mixed vegetables
1 cup small sized dry pasta
1 tsp. sugar
parmesan cheese, finely grated

In a 4-qt. dutch oven, stir together meatballs, broth, beans, tomatoes, and vegetables. Bring to a boil. Stir in pasta. Return to boiling, and then reduce the heat and simmer, uncovered 10 minutes. Stir in sugar. Sprinkle each serving with parmesan cheese.

Bake meatballs at 350 degrees for 25 minutes or until golden. Place 4 meatballs on a skewer. Cook small shelled pasta and toss with a little olive oil and parmesan cheese. Serve alongside the steamed mixed vegetables.

Cornbread

2 cups biscuit mix*
2 eggs
1/3 cup cornmeal
1 cup milk
1 cup sugar
¾ cups oil
½ tsp. baking soda

In a large mixing bowl, beat together liquid ingredients. In a separate bowl, combine dry ingredients. Then combine the two mixtures, and beat until smooth. Bake in a preheated 350 degree oven for 25–30 minutes, until top of cornbread is golden.

*To make your own delicious biscuit mix, combine the following and store in an airtight container in your pantry:

9 cups sifted flour
2 cups shortening
¼ cup sugar
3 Tbsp. baking powder
1 Tbsp. salt

chicken tortilla soup

2 chicken breasts, cooked
1 can whole tomatoes
1 can enchilada sauce
1 medium onion, chopped
1 can green chilies
1 clove garlic, minced
2 cups water
1 can chicken broth
1 tsp. each of cumin, chili powder, and salt
1 bay leaf
1 can corn

Combine all ingredients in a large stock pot, and cook through. Serve with cheese quesadillas and a dollop of sour cream on the soup. A sprinkling of fresh cilantro is also delicious!

vegetable minestrone

2 Tbsp. olive oil
2 cloves garlic, minced
1 medium onion
2 carrots, sliced
2 cups celery, sliced
1 can kidney beans
2 cups cabbage, shredded
1 zucchini, sliced
1 can tomatoes
4 cups chicken broth
1 Tbsp. parsley
½ cup small pasta
2 tsp. basil
1 tsp. oregano, salt, pepper

In a medium saucepan, heat olive oil, and then sauté garlic, onion, carrots, and celery until tender. Add beans, cabbage, zucchini, tomatoes, and chicken broth. Simmer 30 minutes. Add parsley, pasta, basil, and other spices. Serve immediately.

clam chowder

2 cups potatoes, cubed
1 cup onions, chopped
1 cup celery, chopped
2 cans minced clams
1 grated carrot
¾ cups butter
¾ cups flour
1 quart half-and-half
½ tsp. sugar
salt and pepper to taste
2 Tbsp. vinegar

Place potatoes, onion, celery, and clam juice in a large saucepan. Cover all the vegetables with water, and cook 15 minutes or until vegetables are tender. Meanwhile, in a medium saucepan, melt the butter, then add the flour to form a roux. Slowly pour in the half-and-half, sugar, salt and pepper, vinegar, and clams. Stir until thick. Pour mixture into vegetable pot. Stir all together and simmer 10 more minutes. Serve in bread bowls or with French bread and a salad.

taco soup

1 lb. hamburger, browned
1/3 onion
1 can tomato sauce
1 can corn
1 can tomatoes, diced
2 cans kidney beans
1 pkg. taco seasoning mix
Frito chips
cheddar cheese, shredded

Combine all ingredients except chips and cheese. Simmer 25 minutes. Just before serving, pile on the Frito chips and some shredded cheddar cheese.

chunky bacon potato soup

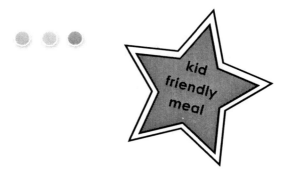

6 slices smoked bacon
1 onion, diced
1 stalk celery, diced
1 can chicken broth
10 potatoes, peeled and cubed
4 tsp. flour
1 pkg. ranch dressing mix*
2 cups half-and-half cream
1 cup sour cream
salt and pepper to taste
2 cups shredded cheddar cheese
¼ cup chopped green onion

Cook and crumble bacon; set aside, reserving the drippings. Stir in onions and celery and cook 5 minutes. Add broth and potatoes and bring to a boil. Simmer until tender.

Mash about ⅓ of the potatoes. In a large bowl, combine flour and ranch mix. Whisk in the half-and-half and sour cream, mixing well. Slowly whisk this mixture into the soup, adding salt and pepper to taste. Top each serving with bacon crumbles, shredded cheese, and green onion.

*To make your own ranch dressing mix, combine the ingredients on the following page and place in an airtight container on your pantry shelf. To make fresh ranch dressing, simply add 3 Tbsp. of ranch dressing mix to 1 cup sour cream and 1 Tbsp. of milk.

Ranch Dressing

1 cup dehydrated milk or buttermilk
6 Tbsp. onion powder
3 Tbsp. garlic powder
3 Tbsp. parsley, crushed
1 Tbsp. beef soup base
1 Tbsp. chicken soup base
1 Tbsp. black pepper
1 Tbsp. celery seed
1 Tbsp. dehydrated cheese

Kid-Friendly Recipe: Bake some potatoes in the oven at 350 until soft. Then top with melted cheese, bacon, and a little ranch dressing if desired.

broccoli cheese soup
in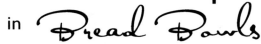

4 bread bowls from the local bakery
3 Tbsp. butter
2 Tbsp. finely chopped onion
3 Tbsp. flour
1/8 tsp. white pepper
1/2 tsp. each salt, thyme, garlic powder
2 cups chicken broth
2 cups milk
1 cup cooked broccoli, finely chopped
2 cups cheddar cheese, shredded

In a sauce pan, sauté butter and onion until soft. Add flour, pepper, salt, thyme, and garlic powder. Stir 3–4 minutes. Slowly add chicken broth until the mixture thickens. Then add in milk, broccoli, and cheese. Simmer 10 minutes. When ready to serve, ladle into soup bowls, and garnish with parsley.

french onion soup

2 thick slices French baguette
butter, softened
2 Tbsp. vegetable oil
1 onion, cut into thin strips
1 red onion, cut into thin strips
1 clove garlic, minced
1 tsp. chopped fresh thyme
1 bunch green onion cut into 1-inch pieces
salt and white pepper to taste
½ cup dry sherry
1 can beef broth
1 can chicken broth
3 Tbsp. cornstarch
2 Tbsp. butter, softened
2 cups Gruyere cheese, shredded

Preheat oven to 350 degrees. Butter baguette slices on both sides. Bake on a baking sheet for 5-7 minutes. Set aside. Heat oil in a large saucepan over medium heat.

Saute white and red onions for about 20 minutes or until caramelized, stirring occasionally. Add garlic, thyme, green onions, salt, and white pepper. Cook 2 minutes. Add sherry to the saucepan, and cook until almost dry.

Add the broths, and bring to a boil. Combine cornstarch and 2 tablespoons butter in a small bowl, stirring to mix well. Add to the soup and stir until butter mixture is melted and soup is thickened slightly.

Remove from heat. Ladle into soup bowls and cover with baguettes and cheese. Place the bowls on a baking sheet and bake for about 10 minutes or until cheese is golden brown and bubbly.

red bean
and Beef Borsht

3 large beets
8 cups beef broth
1 large onion, chopped
1 Tbsp. butter
3 cups shredded green cabbage
4 tsp. lemon juice
1½ cups red kidney beans or small red beans
salt and pepper to taste
sour cream for topping

Wash and peel beets. Grate them coarsely. Bring broth to a boil in a large soup pot. Add chopped onion and beets to the boiling broth. Cook 20 minutes. Add cabbage and beans. Cook another 10 minutes. Add butter, lemon juice, salt, and pepper. Simmer until ready to serve. Serve with a dollop of sour cream and a sprig of fresh parsley. Delicious served with crusty sourdough bread.

pasta and chickpea soup

½ cup olive oil
6 cloves garlic, smashed
1 (19-oz.) can chickpeas, rinsed and drained
salt and pepper to taste
4 cups chicken broth
½ lb. small pasta shells
¾ cup fresh grated parmesan cheese

In a saucepan, sauté garlic in oil 2 minutes. Add chickpeas, salt, and pepper. Stir 3 more minutes. Add broth and bring to a boil. Reduce heat and simmer, covered for 20 minutes.

herbed corn chowder

2 slices bacon, chopped
1 potato, peeled, cubed
2 cups milk
1 cup corn, frozen or fresh
1 onion, chopped
½ red bell pepper, chopped
1 (15-oz.) can creamed corn
1 Tbsp. fresh thyme, chopped

Cook bacon in a heavy saucepan for 3 minutes. Add onion and cook until tender, about 8 minutes. Add potato and bell pepper, and sauté 1 minute more. Add milk and bring to a boil. Reduce heat and simmer until vegetables are tender and soup thickens slightly, stirring occasionally, about 15 minutes. Add corn and 1 tablespoon fresh thyme, or ½ tsp. dried thyme. Season with salt and pepper to taste.

cauliflower and Blue Cheese Soup

2 stalks celery, chopped
1 large onion, chopped
2 cloves garlic, minced
1 Tbsp. olive oil
5 cups chicken stock
1 head cauliflower, chopped
1/3 cup white wine
1 Tbsp. lemon juice
1 tsp. Worcestershire sauce
1/4 tsp. dried thyme
1 pinch fried marjoram
dash of hot pepper sauce
1 cup crumbled blue cheese
2 1/2 cups milk
1/2 cup flour

In a Dutch oven, sauté celery, onion, and garlic in oil. Stir in stock, cauliflower, white wine, lemon juice, Worcestershire sauce, thyme, marjoram, and hot pepper sauce. Bring to a boil over high heat. Reduce heat. Cover and simmer 15 minutes or until cauliflower is tender. Remove vegetables and puree in blender. Stir vegetables back into pot. Stir in blue cheese. Whisk flour into pot. Stir in milk. Bring to almost boiling. Reduce heat and cook until thickened, adding more milk to thin if necessary.

cheese tortellini soup

2 slices cooked bacon, chopped
1/3 cup chopped onion
2 cloves garlic, minced
4 cups chicken broth
3 cups frozen cheese-filled tortellini (12 oz.)
1 (10-oz.) package frozen spinach
ground black pepper
parmesan cheese shavings

In a large saucepan, cook bacon over medium-high heat about 3 minutes or until crisp. Add onion; cook 3 minutes more. Stir in garlic; cook 1 minute more. Add broth; bring to boiling. Stir in tortellini. Return package directions, adding spinach for the last 3 minutes of cooking time. Season to taste with pepper, and if desired, garnish with parmesan cheese.

chicken noodle and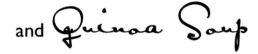

3 chicken breasts
1 onion, chopped
2 stalks celery
2 garlic cloves, chopped
2 quarts water
1 Tbsp. salt
2 tsp. pepper
2 carrots, sliced

Place all ingredients except carrots in electric pressure cooker and pressure on high 14 minutes. Remove the lid and strain the liquid off of the chicken, saving the liquid. Discard cooked vegetables. Place liquid back in pressure cooker, and shred the chicken, adding back into the broth. Add the sliced carrots as well as the following ingredients:

1 cup uncooked white quinoa
1 lb. egg noodles
1 quart more water

Pressure for 6 minutes. Garnish with chopped parsley.

autumn harvest Split Pea Soup

1¼ cups dried split peas
4 cups water
¼ cup chopped shallots
½ cup chopped carrots
2 stalks celery, sliced
1 bay leaf
1 tsp. salt
½ tsp. garlic
¼ tsp. pepper
8 oz. cream cheese

In a medium saucepan, cook dried split peas, shallots, carrots, celery, and bay leaf in 4 cups water for 35 minutes. Add garlic, salt, and pepper. Simmer 10 more minutes. Puree vegetable mixture in a blender until smooth, and then return to the pot. Just before serving, mix in cream cheese, until melted and creamy. Serve with warm bread.

garden vegetable Taboulleh Stew

1 large onion, chopped
2 medium carrots, sliced
1 cup green beans, cut into 1-inch sections
2 medium green onions, sliced
1 can chick peas, rinsed and drained
2 cans diced tomatoes
salt and pepper to taste
1 box Taboulleh mix
1½ cups water
¼ cup olive oil
sour cream
fresh mint

Layer ingredients in slow cooker in this order: onion, carrots, green beans, green onions, zucchini, chick peas, tomatoes with juice, salt, and pepper. Sprinkle mix over vegetables. Pour water and olive oil evenly over top. Cover and cook in Crock-Pot on low 6 hours, or until vegetables are tender-crisp. Garnish with sour cream and fresh mint.

navy bean and Bacon Chowder

3 cups white beans, rinsed, drained
6 slices thick bacon
1 medium carrot and celery stalk, chopped
1 cup milk
1 medium onion, chopped
1 small turnip, chopped
1 tsp. dried Italian seasoning
1 large can chicken broth

Cook bacon and drain. Place all ingredients except milk in slow cooker. Cook 8 hours on low. Process soup with milk in a blender, and heat through.

ravioli and cabbage soup

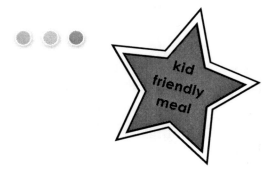

5 slices bacon
1 small onion, chopped
2 cloves garlic, minced
1 Tbsp. chopped parsley
8 cups beef stock
2 cups water
2 cups shredded cabbage
1 carrot, thinly sliced
1 lb. frozen ravioli
parmesan cheese

Cut bacon into ½-inch pieces. Cook until done. Spoon off all but 2 Tbsp. drippings. Add onion, garlic, and parsley, and cook until onion and bacon are browned. Add stock, water, cabbage, and carrot. Bring to a boil gently, uncovered, stirring occasionally, until ravioli are just tender. Sprinkle with parmesan cheese.

Kid-Friendly Recipe: Cook the ravioli briefly in boiling salt water, and set aside. Meanwhile, make a simple white sauce using the recipe on page 93. Pour over cooked ravioli, sprinkle with bacon. Serve with parmesan bread. To make the bread, spread sourdough bread with a little butter and garlic, then sprinkle with parmesan cheese. Grill in the oven just until golden.

SALADS

Chick Pea and Vegetable Salad 64
Honey Lime Quinoa Pasta Salad 65
Bulgur Wheat Salad with Garlic Parsley Pita 66
Southwestern Layer Salad 67
Mango Chicken Salad 68
Spinach Chicken Salad 69
Asian Cabbage Salad 70
Couscous Salad 71
Strawberry Wonton Chicken Salad 72
Wheat Berry, Chicken, and Pasta Salad 73
Layered Spinach Salad 74
Asian Chicken Pasta Salad 75
Brazilian Pork Salad 76
Steak and Pepper Salad 77
Broccoli Cashew Salad 78
Turkey Red Grape Salad 79
Spinach Salad 80
Festive Chicken Salad 81
Shrimp, Avocado, and Noodle Salad 82
Black Bean, Barley, and Pine Nut Salad 84

chick pea and Vegetable Salad

1½ lbs. baby red potatoes, halved
1 cup grape tomatoes, halved
2 cups cooked chickpeas, drained and rinsed*
¾ cups walnut halves
2 Tbsp. rice wine vinegar
1 Tbsp. Dijon mustard
¼ cup olive oil
pinch of sugar
8 oz. fresh young asparagus spears, trimmed
salt and pepper to taste
6 large scallions, trimmed to just above the white part
10 oz. baby spinach leaves

Combine rice vinegar, mustard, olive oil, and sugar in a small bowl and whisk well. Cook potatoes in a small saucepan until almost done. Add asparagus for the last 3 minutes of cooking. Drain potatoes and asparagus well. Rinse under cold running water, and rinse again.

Dice potatoes, slice scallions, and add chickpeas. Pour dressing over salad and toss well.

Add salt and pepper to taste. Place baby spinach in a large, flat salad bowl, and top with the vegetable mixture.

*Canned chickpeas can also be used.

honey lime Quinoa Pasta Salad

    3 cups small shell pasta, cooked
    1 cup red quinoa, cooked and drained*
    1 can pineapple tidbits, drained
    ½ cup celery, chopped
    ¼ cup green onion, sliced
    1 Gala apple, chopped
    1 cup cheddar cheese, grated

In a large salad bowl, combine all these ingredients. Then mix in honey lime dressing and serve immediately.

    1 cup mayonnaise
    ¼ cup cream cheese, softened
    3 Tbsp. lime juice
    3 Tbsp. honey
    1 Tbsp. Dijon mustard
    salt and pepper to taste

Combine all ingredients in a food processor, and mix until smooth.

*To cook quinoa, place ½ cup quinoa and 2 cups water in a small saucepan. Bring to a boil, and then cover the pan and reduce the heat to simmer. Cook 25 minutes or until quinoa is al dente. Drain excess water and rinse.

bulgur wheat salad with Garlic Parsley Pita

1 cup diced fresh tomatoes
4 cups each Romaine and iceberg lettuce
1 cup diced fresh cucumbers
¼ cup green onions, sliced thin
½ cup fresh minced parsley
½ cup fresh minced mint
1 cup prepared bulgur wheat
Brianna's vinaigrette with strawberry on the cover

Combine all ingredients together in a large salad bowl and toss. This can be eaten alone, or stuffed in a pita pocket with grated cheese and a drizzle of plain yogurt.

Garlic Parsley Pita

3–4 cups flour
1 tsp. salt
1 Tbsp. yeast
1 Tbsp. oil
¼ tsp. sugar

1¹/₃ cups warm water
1 tsp. crushed fresh garlic
2 Tbsp. fresh parsley, chopped

In a large mixing bowl, combine yeast, sugar, warm water, oil, and salt. Add 2 cups flour, adding more as needed to make a soft and elastic dough. Add in the parsley and the garlic, and knead 6 minutes. Divide dough into 8 sections. On a heavily floured countertop, roll each ball into flat circles, and allow to rise 40 minutes, covered with a dish towel. Preheat oven and baking sheet to 500 degrees. Carefully transfer pita rounds onto the baking tray, baking 3 at a time. Remove when slightly golden. Cut in 2.

southwestern layer salad

8 cups Romaine, shredded
8 hard boiled eggs, sliced
3½ cups cherry tomatoes, quartered
2 cans whole kernel corn
1 can black beans, drained
½ cup green onions, sliced
2 medium avocados, peeled, diced
1 can sliced olives
2 cups shredded cheddar cheese

Dressing

1½ cups mayonnaise
½ tsp. cumin
²/₃ cups salsa
½ tsp. chili powder
2 Tbsp. lime juice
1¼ cups minced cilantro

In a glass bowl, layer all ingredients of the salad, with the egg slices lining the sides of the bowl. Mix dressing ingredients together, and pour on just before serving.

mango chicken salad

 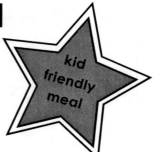

1 head Romaine lettuce
3 tomatoes, diced
½ cup feta cheese
1 mango, diced
2 chicken breasts, cooked and seasoned with lemon pepper
1 Tbsp. sesame seeds
1 bag tortilla chips
2 cups warm cooked rice

Dressing

¼ cup Dijon mustard
2 Tbsp. lime juice
1 tsp. chili powder
¾ cups mayonnaise
½ cup white vinegar
¼ cup soy sauce
½ cup white sugar
2 Tbsp. minced garlic
2 Tbsp. ginger powder

Combine all salad ingredients together in a large bowl. Then combine all dressing ingredients together, and mix until smooth. Dress the salad, and serve immediately.

Kid-Friendly Recipe: Make sure the mango is ripe enough to be sweet. Slice the mango in 4 large wedges, and lay the wedges end to end in a square on the child's plate. In the center of the square, scoop some steamed and buttered rice, chopped chicken, a few broken tortilla chips, and a little shredded cheese. Drizzle with a little of the salad dressing you prepared.

spinach chicken salad

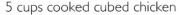

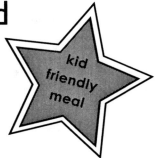

5 cups cooked cubed chicken
2 cups green grapes
1 cup fresh snow peas
2 cups spinach
2 cups sliced celery
7 oz. corkscrew pasta
1 jar artichoke hearts
1 large cucumber, sliced
3 green onions, sliced
2 cans mandarin oranges

Dressing

1½ cups vegetable oil
¼ cup sugar
2 Tbsp. white wine vinegar
1 tsp. salt
½ tsp. dried minced onion
1 tsp. lemon juice
2 Tbsp. fresh parsley, minced

Combine all salad ingredients in a large bowl. In a separate bowl, mix together dressing ingredients. Dress salad just before serving. Serve with warm breadsticks.

Kid-Friendly Recipe: Make the kids delicious skewers by threading chunks of cucumber, grapes, oranges, and grilled chicken on a stick. Serve with pasta and basil butter. (See page 6 for the basil butter recipe.)

asian cabbage salad

 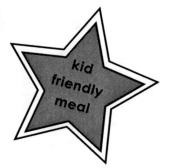

4 chicken breasts
Yoshida's Gourmet Sauce
¼ cup almonds, sliced
6 green onions, sliced
2 carrots, shredded
1 small head cabbage
2 pkgs. chicken ramen noodles

In a pressure cooker, combine 4 chicken breasts with ½ bottle of Yoshida's Gourmet Sauce. (This can also be done in the oven, but it may take twice as long to cook.) Cook chicken until it shreds easily. Then set chicken aside to cool. In a small skillet, place ¼ cup almonds and 1 tablespoon sugar. Carmelize almonds and allow them to cool. In a large salad bowl, combine chicken, sliced onions, shredded carrots, shredded cabbage, and 2 packages ramen noodles, broken apart. Reserve the flavor packets for the dressing.

Dressing
¾ cups canola oil
sesame seeds
6 Tbsp. rice vinegar
4 Tbsp. sugar
1 chicken flavor ramen seasoning packet

Dress the salad just before serving. This is delicious served with fresh cornbread.

Kid-Friendly Recipe: Cook the ramen as usual. Just before serving, add a few small chicken dices. Serve some baby carrots and a few whole almonds on the side.

couscous salad

2 cups chicken stock
½ tsp. each ginger, cumin, curry
¾ tsp. cinnamon
1 medium carrot, diced
1 cup couscous, uncooked
1 small red onion, diced
1 small red bell pepper, diced into ¼-inch pieces
1 granny smith apple, diced
⅛ cup currants or raisins
½ cup cooked garbanzo beans
½ cup cooked lentils
¼ cup fresh lemon juice
½ tsp. salt
¼ tsp. fresh ground pepper

In a heavy medium saucepan, whisk together the stock, cinnamon, ginger, cumin, and curry. Add couscous in a slow, steady stream, stirring constantly, and continue to boil, stirring, for 1 minute. Cover the pot tightly, remove from the heat, and let stand for 15 minutes. Transfer couscous to large bowl and allow to cool, fluffing with a fork occasionally. Add the rest of the ingredients and toss well. Allow to sit refrigerated several hours before serving.

strawberry wonton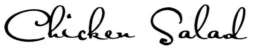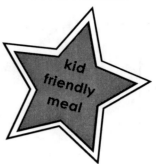

15 square wonton wrappers, cut into thin strips, fried
1 pkg. fresh baby spinach
1 large head Romaine, washed and torn
½ cup red bell pepper, chop
½ red onion, chopped
1 cup strawberries, sliced
½ cup sliced almonds
½ cup bacon, cooked, chop
2-3 chicken breasts, cooked, chopped, and seasoned with Montreal seasoning.

Dressing

¼ cup red wine vinegar
⅓ cup oil
¼ tsp. salt
3 Tbsp. sugar
½ tsp. dry mustard
½ cup strawberry jam.

Combine all salad ingredients, and then all the dressing ingredients, and mix to coat. Delicious with garlic and parmesan breadsticks.

Kid-Friendly Recipe: Tear the Romaine and spinach into bite-size pieces and top with pieces of bacon. Grill chicken chunks seasoned with lemon pepper, and put on a skewer alternating with whole strawberries. Serve with a raspberry vinaigrette dip.

wheat berry, chicken, and Pasta Salad

4 cups cooked, cubed chicken breasts
1 stalk celery, thinly sliced
2 cups diced granny smith apples
½ cup cooked wheat berries
8 oz. corkscrew pasta, cooked, drained
½ cup seedless grapes, halved
1 (8-oz.) can pineapple tidbits

Combine all ingredients in a salad bowl, and make the dressing below. Toss together and allow to chill 4 hours to combine flavors. Serve on a bed of lettuce.

Dressing

1 cup mayonnaise
$1/3$ cup sour cream
1 tsp. lime zest
3 Tbsp. lime juice
2 Tbsp. honey
2 tsp. grated ginger
¼ tsp. salt

layered spinach salad

1 pkg. frozen peas
8 oz. bacon, crumbled
1 bag torn spinach
4 scallions, chopped
4 hard boiled eggs, shelled, sliced
1 can water chestnuts
1 bottle ranch dressing
½ cup grated parmesan
2 Tbsp. fresh chopped parsley

Layer spinach, eggs, bacon, scallions, peas, and chestnuts in that order in a 4 qt. glass serving bowl. Pour dressing over salad, and then sprinkle parmesan and parsley on top. Cover bowl with plastic, and chill for at least an hour, but preferably overnight.

asian chicken
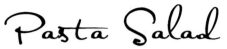

- 1 small pkg. spinach
- 8 oz. bowtie pasta
- 2–4 Tbsp. sesame seeds for topping
- ½ cup sunflower seeds
- 3 chicken breasts, cubed
- 1 tsp. lemon pepper
- 1 cup bean sprouts

Season chicken with lemon pepper and cook until done. Combine all ingredients in a salad bowl. Cover until ready to serve, and then add the dressing below:

Dressing

- ½ cup oil
- ½ cup sugar
- 1 tsp. salt
- 1 tsp. sesame seeds
- 3 Tbsp. soy sauce
- 2 Tbsp. rice vinegar
- ½ tsp. sesame oil
- 1 tsp. fresh garlic, minced

Mix well in a blender. Pour on pasta salad when ready to serve. Great served along with parmesan breadsticks.

brazilian pork salad
and Tangerine Vinaigrette

1½ lbs. pork tenderloin, cut into thin strips
1 medium bunch kale
2 tsp. ground coriander, divided
¼ tsp. salt
¼ tsp. white pepper
2 Tbsp. olive oil
1 can black beans, rinsed, drained
¼ cup lime juice
⅓ cup tangerine juice
1 tsp. red pepper flakes
1¼ cups fresh pineapple chunks, divided
½ cup fresh cilantro
4 tangerines, peeled and divided
3 Tbsp. shredded toasted coconut

Stack kale leaves and roll crosswise into very thin strips. Place in serving bowl. Season pork strips with 1 teaspoon coriander, salt, and pepper. Heat 1 tablespoon olive oil in a nonstick skillet over high heat.

Stir fry pork strips until they are nicely brown, about 3–5 minutes. Place strips in a serving dish with black beans and kale. In a blender, combine citrus juices, the remaining tablespoon olive oil, red pepper flakes, cilantro, and salt and pepper. Blend until smooth. Add tangerine sections and pineapple to the salad. Toss salad with dressing. Garnish with coconut.

steak and pepper salad

olive oil
1 red pepper, sliced thin
1 yellow pepper, sliced thin
1 sweet onion, sliced thin
12 oz. beef sirloin steak, cut in thin strips
1 tsp. salt
1 can red kidney beans, rinsed, drained
¼ tsp. pepper
3 Tbsp. balsamic vinegar
2 Tbsp. Worcestershire sauce
½ tsp. sugar
2 cups torn Romaine leaves
2 cups torn iceberg lettuce leaves

Put about 1 tablespoon olive oil in a large nonstick skillet over medium high heat. Add peppers and cook, stirring, just until tender-crisp. Stir in onion, until onion is browned and peppers are tender. Remove vegetables and set aside in a bowl. Sprinkle steak with the salt. In the same skillet, add another 1 tablespoon olive oil and cook steak about 5 minutes on each side. Add kidney beans to the drippings and cook just until beans are warm. Spoon over steak and peppers and remove skillet from heat. Combine black pepper, vinegar, Worcestershire, and sugar; add to the skillet. Add another 2 tablespoons of olive oil to the skillet mixture and blend well. Place lettuce in a large salad bowl and top with the bean, steak, and pepper mixture. Drizzle the warm dressing over the salad. Toss to serve.

broccoli cashew salad
and Oatmeal Rolls

1 lb. bacon, cooked
1 cup mayonnaise
2 lbs. fresh broccoli, broken into florets
½ cup raisins
2 tsp. cider vinegar
1 cup roasted cashews
½ cup white sugar
¼ cup red onion, finely chopped

Whisk together mayonnaise, cider vinegar, and sugar in a mixing bowl until sugar has dissolved. Add broccoli, raisins, cashews, onion, and crumbled bacon. Stir until evenly coated. Cover and refrigerate salad for at least 2 hours. Let stand at room temperature 15 to 20 minutes before serving.

Oatmeal Rolls

2⅓ cups water, divided
1 cup oats
⅔ cups brown sugar
3 Tbsp. butter
1½ tsp. salt
2 Tbsp. yeast
5 cup flour

Bring 2 cups water to a boil. Add oats. Cook 10 minutes. Add rest of the water, brown sugar, butter, salt and 2 cups flour. Mix until smooth. Add yeast and the rest of the flour to form a soft elastic dough. Rise 1 hour. Make 24 balls and place in a 9x13 pan. Rise ½ hour longer, and bake at 350 degrees for 20–25 minutes, until lightly golden.

turkey red grape salad

1 (8-oz.) pkg. mostaccioli pasta
1½ cups mayonnaise
2 cups halved seedless red grapes
2 cups diced turkey
1 cup sour cream
1 cup chopped celery
1 head Romaine lettuce, torn
1 cup spinach, torn
slivered almonds

Bring a large pot of lightly salted water to a boil. Add pasta, and cook 8–10 minutes, or until tender. Drain and run under cold water to cool. Drain again, and transfer to a large bowl. In a separate bowl, stir together mayonnaise, sour cream, and slivered almonds.

spinach salad

with *Avocado, Oranges, and Feta*

kid friendly meal

1/3 cup rice vinegar
3 Tbsp. sugar
1 tsp. salt
1/2 tsp. pepper
1/2 tsp. sesame oil
1/2 cup vegetable oil
6 oz. spinach leaves
1 head Romaine, washed and torn
1/2 cup dried cranberries
1/2 cup pecans, toasted and chopped
4–8 oz. crumbled feta
1–2 avocados, cubed
1 can mandarin oranges
1/2 red onion, sliced

Mix together vinegar, sugar, salt, sesame oil, pepper, and vegetable oil in a small bowl. Toss the spinach and Romaine together in a salad bowl. Top the greens with all the other ingredients, and drizzle with salad dressing. Serve with multi-grain crackers.

Kid-Friendly Recipe: Make a simple salad of spinach leaves, craisins, orange slices, and your child's favorite dressing. You may want to bake the crackers topped with a sprinkle of powdered cheddar cheese.

festive chicken salad
in Pastry Puff Shell

• • •

Chicken Salad

    2 chicken breasts, shredded or cubed
    ¼ cup mayonnaise
    8 oz. cream cheese
    2 green onions, sliced
    ¼ cup pineapple tidbits
    1 stalk celery, sliced
    slivered almonds
    salt and pepper to taste
    lemon juice

In a medium bowl, combine the cooked chicken cubes, green onions, sliced celery, pineapple tidbits, and slivered almonds. In a smaller bowl, combine the softened cream cheese, mayonnaise, salt and pepper to taste, and a dash of lemon juice. Combine both mixtures until well incorporated. Stuff inside pastry puff shells.

Pastry Puff Shells:

    1½ cups biscuit mix
    2 cups water
    4 eggs

In a small saucepan, bring water to a boil. Add biscuit mix all at once and stir vigorously until a soft ball forms. Continue cooking 2 minutes. Transfer ball to a mixing bowl, and beat in eggs, one at a time, until gluey and thick dough forms. Line baking sheet with a piece of parchment paper, and spoon the dough by 2 tablespoons full onto the baking sheet. Bake at 400 for 10 minutes, and then reduce heat to 350 degrees. Bake about 20 minutes, until lightly golden and no water beads appear on the puffs. Cool completely. Cut off the tops, and fill with chicken salad.

shrimp, avocado, and noodle salad with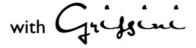

3 quarts water
12 large shrimp, peeled, deveined
4 oz. Asian rice-stick noodles, softened in hot water (about 15 minutes)
3 green onions, thinly sliced diagonally
1 large carrot, peeled, julienned
Honey Ginger Dressing (below)
salt and pepper to taste
1 firm avocado

Bring water to a boil and simmer shrimp just until cooked through. Set aside. Return water to a boil, and add softened noodles. Cook noodles for 2 minutes or just until tender. Rinse noodles in a colander under cold water to stop the cooking process; drain well. Cut noodles with scissors into 4-inch lengths. Gently toss the shrimp, noodles, onions, carrot, and honey ginger dressing in a bowl. Season with salt and pepper. Just before serving, pit and peel the avocado, cut into ½-inch pieces, and place on top of the salad.

Honey Ginger Dressing

1 Tbsp. honey
1 Tbsp. fresh lemon juice
1½ tsp. peeled minced fresh ginger
2 Tbsp. vegetable oil
salt and pepper to taste

Whisk together the honey, lemon juice, and ginger in a small bowl. Add oil in a slow stream, whisking until well blended. Season with salt and pepper.

Grissini

Grissini is simply a long skinny breadstick—light and delicious, and full of flavor. I like to serve grissini in a tall glass vase for a little extra pizzazz!

- 2 ½ tsp. yeast
- ½ tsp. sugar
- 1½ cups warm water
- 3 Tbsp. olive oil
- 1½ tsp. salt
- 1½ tsp. dried rosemary
- ½ cup cornmeal or semolina flour
- 3–3 ½ cups white flour

Dissolve yeast in ½ cup warm water and sugar for 5 minutes. In an electric mixer, combine the rest of the water, oil, salt, rosemary, semolina flour, and 1 cup white flour. Beat on medium speed about 1 minute until creamy. Add the yeast mixture and 1 cup of white flour and beat another minute. Keep adding flour until dough comes away from the bowl and is smooth and elastic, about 4 minutes. Sprinkle a board with semolina flour and pat or roll the dough into a 14x8 inch rectangle. Brush surface with oil. Cover loosely with plastic wrap and let rise on the board at room temperature until doubled in bulk, 1–1½ hours.

Place a baking stone on the center oven rack and preheat to 375 degrees. Line three baking sheets with parchment paper and brush the paper with oil. Rub the surface of the dough with a few tablespoons of semolina flour. With a sharp knife, cut the dough crosswise into 4 equal portions. One at a time, cut each portion lengthwise into 8 strips. Pick up the end of each strip and stretch and roll out the width of a prepared sheet. Place the strips ½ inch apart on the sheets. One at a time, place the sheets on the stone and bake until the bread sticks are lightly browned and crisp, 16–22 minutes. Transfer to racks to cool completely.

black bean, barley, and Pine Nut Salad

1 cup barley
6 Tbsp. lemon juice
1 Tbsp. Dijon mustard
salt and pepper to taste
¾ cups olive oil
3 cups black beans, rinsed
½ cup finely chopped red onion and drained
1 lb. raw green beans, trimmed and cut into ¼-inch pieces
½ cup pine nuts, toasted

Combine barley with 4 cups boiling salted water and simmer, covered for 45 minutes or until cooked but still al dente. Drain barley, rinse, and drain well again. In a small bowl, combine lemon juice, mustard, salt, and pepper. Add oil in a thin stream, whisking as you add until dressing is thickened. In a larger bowl, combine the beans, barley, and onion. Pour dressing over the bean mixture and toss until well mixed. In a saucepan of boiling water, cook the green beans for 4–5 minutes until tender-crisp; drain and rinse immediately under cold water. Add the green beans and pine nuts to the black bean mixture and toss well once more. Serve chilled or at room temperature.

SANDWICHES/ WRAPS

Stroganoff Sandwiches 86
Chicken Hummus Wraps 87
Hoagie Sandwiches 88
Veggie Cheese Paninis 89

stroganoff sandwiches

1 lb. lean ground beef
½ onion, chopped*
2 cups sour cream
2 Tbsp. Worcestershire sauce
crushed garlic and garlic powder
salt and pepper to taste
1 green pepper, chopped
2 tomatoes, sliced
cheddar cheese
1 loaf French bread

Brown hamburger with onion and drain. Add all other ingredients except tomatoes, cheese, and bread. Cut bread horizontally and put on a cookie sheet. Spread meat mixture on both lengths of bread. Put sliced tomatoes on top and smother with cheese. Bake at 350 degrees until cheese is melted.

*Substitute 2 tablespoons chopped dehydrated onion if desired and sauté with meat.

chicken and hummus wraps

You can either use hummus from the supermarket, or try mine, homemade!

Hummus

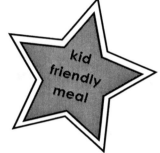

    1 cup garbanzo beans, cooked and drained
    1 clove garlic, minced
    3 Tbsp. lemon or lime juice
    ¼ cup olive oil
    1 Tbsp. parsley, chopped
    sea salt and pepper to taste

Combine all ingredients in a blender until smooth, adding a little water if necessary. Then put your wraps together:

    1 cup hummus or vegetable cream cheese spread
    4 10-inch flour tortillas
    ½ cup plain yogurt or sour cream
    1 cup cooked chicken breast
    ¾ cups Roma tomatoes, chopped
    ¾ cups thin sliced cucumber

Spread hummus evenly over tortillas; spread yogurt or sour cream over hummus. Top with shredded chicken, tomatoes, and cucumber. Roll up tortillas. Makes 4 wraps.

Kid-Friendly Recipe: Spread a thin layer of cream cheese over the tortillas, and serve the hummus dip on the side. Serve with slices of tomato and cucumber on the side.

hoagie sandwiches

1 loaf French bread, cut lengthwise in half
8 oz. softened cream cheese
3 Tbsp. mayonnaise
ham, turkey, roast beef
Swiss cheese slices
lettuce, shredded
tomato slices
red onion, sliced

Zesty Italian Dressing

Spread each side of the French bread loaves with softened cream cheese. On the bottom half of the French bread loaf, layer ham, turkey, roast beef, Swiss cheese, lettuce, tomato, and red onion. Then sprinkle with zesty Italian dressing and top with the other side of the French bread loaf.

Wrap the loaf tightly with plastic wrap and allow to sit two hours in the fridge before serving. Serve with an assortment of chips and some fresh fruit.

veggie cheese paninis
and Tomato Soup

8 ½-inch-thick slices of hearty bread
4 tsp. olive oil
2 Tbsp. honey mustard or ranch dressing
4 ounces cheddar cheese
½ cup cucumber or Roma tomatoes, thinly sliced
½ cup fresh spinach
¼ cup red pepper, thinly sliced
4 cups canned tomato soup
1 cup chopped Roma tomatoes
1 Tbsp. balsamic vinegar
½ cup sour cream

Brush one side of bread slices lightly with oil. Brush the other side of bread slices with honey mustard. Top the mustard sides of four of the bread slices with cheese. Top cheese with cucumber, spinach, and red pepper. Top with remaining bread slices, mustard sides down. Preheat panini press and place the sandwiches on the grill. Grill about 3 minutes, until golden. Cut each sandwich in half. Meanwhile, in a medium sauce pan, stir together canned tomato soup, Roma tomatoes, vinegar, and sour cream. Warm through and serve with paninis.

PIZZA/PASTA

Pasta Fagioli 92
Tomato Alfredo 93
Barbecue Chicken Pizza 94
Stuffed Shells 96
Spaghetti and Meatballs 97
Chicken Caesar Salad Pizza 98
Lemon Shrimp and
    Spinach Linguini 99
Chicken Parmesan 100
Pasta with Shrimp,
    Asparagus, and Tomatoes 102
Pesto Pizza and Artichokes 103
Chicken Lasagna Rolls 104

pasta fagioli

 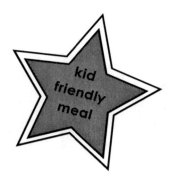

2 Tbsp. olive oil
1 clove minced garlic
1 large onion, chopped
1 8 oz. can tomato sauce
1 tsp. salt, 1 tsp. pepper
2 tsp. dried basil
2 Tbsp. parsley, chopped
2 cups small shell pasta, cooked
1 can kidney beans
fresh, grated parmesan

Heat olive oil and sauté onion and garlic in a large saucepan. Add the rest of the ingredients, except pasta and parmesan cheese. Simmer for 25 minutes, adding the pasta and parmesan cheese just before serving.

Kid-Friendly Recipe: Using the same small shells, make a delicious homemade mac and cheese using one of my favorite make-ahead pantry mixes—a real cheddar cheese sauce mix.

Cheddar Cheese Sauce Mix

4 ½ cups powdered cheddar Cheese
2 $^2/_3$ cups powdered butter
2 $^2/_3$ cups powdered milk
2 $^2/_3$ cups flour
1 Tbsp. sea salt
2 tsp. onion powder

Store mix in an airtight container in the pantry. To make the cheese sauce, simply combine 1 cup milk or water and ⅓ cup Cheddar Cheese Sauce mix in a small pan, and cook on medium until sauce thickens. Add ½ cup fresh cheddar cheese and a dash of nutmeg if desired. Pour over small cooked shells and enjoy!

Serve this mac and cheese with some carrot sticks and apple slices, and call it a meal!

tomato alfredo
on Angel Hair Pasta

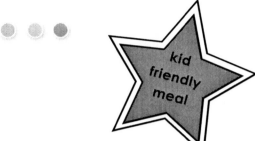

1 can diced tomatoes
1 cup sour cream
¾ cups parmesan cheese
¾ cups frozen peas
1 lb. angel hair pasta
salt and pepper to taste

Cook pasta, adding peas at the end. Drain. Combine other ingredients, and pour over prepared pasta.

Kid-Friendly Recipe: Prepare pasta plain. Meanwhile, prepare a simple white sauce with this all natural mix:

White Sauce Mix

2 cups powdered milk
2 cups powdered butter
2 cups flour
1 Tbsp. salt

Mix all ingredients together and store in an airtight container in the pantry. To make the white sauce, simply combine 1 cup water and ⅓ cup White Sauce Mix in a small pot. Add 2 tablespoons onion soup mix, 1 tsp. parsley, ¼ cup softened cream cheese, and ¼ cup grated parmesan cheese. Mix until thick and smooth, adding more water if desired. Pour over pasta, and serve with a side of cooked peas.

barbecue chicken pizza

I love to bake these pizzas outside on the grill. It gives them a light, smoky flavor. I also like to also bake them as individual pizza rounds on lightly sprayed tin foil.

Pizza Dough

2 cups hot water
2 Tbsp. yeast
sprinkle of sugar
2 cups milk
1 cube butter
¼ cup sugar
2 tsp. salt
⅓ cup oil
2 Tbsp. cardamom

In a small bowl, mix together 2 cups hot water, yeast, and sugar. Allow it to sit 10 minutes. Then add all the other ingredients and mix about 8 minutes, until smooth. Take dough out of the mixer and knead a little olive oil into the dough. Place the dough inside the bowl again, and cover with saran wrap. Let rise 30–60 minutes. Spray squares of tin foil with cooking spray. Load the toppings on each pizza, and then cook pizzas on the grill on low until crust is golden brown. Yield: 24 mini pizzas.

Barbecue Chicken Topping

1 cup ketchup
1 cup water
3 Tbsp. Worcestershire sauce
½ cup brown sugar
2 cups shredded cooked chicken
pineapple tidbits
1 green pepper, diced

In a small saucepan, combine all ingredients but the chicken. Simmer 20 minutes. Then add the shredded cooked chicken. Pour a little sauce on each pizza dough round, and then top with pineapple, sliced green peppers, and shredded mozzarella cheese.

stuffed shells

12 large pasta shells, uncooked
1 cup ricotta
¼ cup shredded parmesan
1 egg
2 Tbsp. parsley, chopped
¼ tsp. garlic salt
½ tsp. salt
⅛ tsp. pepper
1 cup mozzarella cheese, shredded

Pasta Sauce

In a saucepan, bring water to a boil with 1 teaspoon oil. Cook large pasta shells, and drain. Meanwhile, combine ricotta, parmesan, egg, parsley, garlic salt, salt and pepper, and ½ cup mozzarella cheese. Spoon mixture into each of the shells.

In an 8x8 inch baking dish, spoon ½ cup of the pasta sauce on the bottom, placing the filled shells on top. Then spoon another ½ cup of the pasta sauce over the top of the shells, adding more pasta sauce, if you'd like. Sprinkle the rest of the mozzarella cheese on top, and cover with foil. Bake in a 350 degree oven for 25–30 minutes, until the cheese melts and the sauce bubbles. Serve with fresh garlic bread.

spaghetti and meatballs

1 lb. spaghetti
2 cups pasta sauce
2 cups frozen Italian meatballs
fresh parmesan
fresh basil leaves, torn
1 cup fresh sliced mushrooms

Prepare spaghetti according to package directions. Toss with a little olive oil and keep warm. Meanwhile, in a medium saucepan, combine meatballs, pasta sauce, and mushrooms, and allow to simmer 20 minutes. When ready to serve, toss in torn basil leaves and pour sauce over spaghetti. Sprinkle generously with fresh parmesan.

chicken caesar salad pizza

1 pizza crust baked on a ceramic stone and cooled (use my former pizza crust recipe)
½ cup parmesan cheese, grated, and divided
½ cup Caesar dressing
1 tsp. lemon pepper
1 garlic clove, minced
1 pkg. softened cream cheese
3 chicken breasts, cooked
½ red bell pepper, sliced thin and shredded
4 cups Romaine lettuce, thinly sliced
1 can olives

In a small bowl, combine ¼ cup of the cheese, dressing, lemon pepper, and garlic. Place cream cheese in another bowl; add half of the dressing and mix well. Chop half of the chicken and add to cream cheese mixture. Slice remaining chicken into thin strips; slice lettuce and chop bell pepper and slice olives. Place lettuce, bell pepper, and olives in large bowl. Add remaining dressing mixture; toss to coat. Spread cream cheese mixture on crust. Top with salad mixture. Arrange chicken strips over the salad; sprinkle with remaining parmesan cheese. Makes 12 servings.

lemon shrimp and Spinach linguini

1 lb. spinach linguini
½ cup olive oil
zest from one lemon
juice from 2 lemons
½ cup chopped green onion
¼ cup fresh parsley, chopped
salt and pepper to taste
1 cup fresh parmesan cheese
1 bunch of asparagus or green beans

Boil and drain linguini. In a dressing bowl, combine the oil, zest, lemon juice, parsley, and salt and pepper. Mix well. Pour over the pasta, and add the green onion, asparagus, and parmesan cheese. Mix thoroughly. This tastes delicious hot or cold, with some delicious crusty sour dough bread and some sparkling cider!

chicken parmesan over Angel Hair Pasta

This recipe is truly "from scratch," using fresh herbs and homemade marinara sauce. It's truly worth every ounce of work! If you don't have fresh herbs, use ⅓ of the amount asked for and use dried herbs instead. Enjoy!

```
3 Tbsp. olive oil
1 tsp. chopped rosemary
1 tsp. chopped thyme
1 tsp. chopped parsley
salt and pepper to taste
8 chicken cutlets (3 oz. each)
1½ cups Simple Marinara Sauce (see next page)
½ cup mozzarella cheese, shredded
16 tsp. grated parmesan
2 Tbsp. butter
```

Preheat oven to 500 degrees. Stir the oil and herbs in a small bowl to blend. Season with salt and pepper. Brush both sides of the cutlets with the herb oil. Heat a heavy large oven-proof skillet over high heat. Add cutlets and cook just until brown, about 2 minutes per side. Remove skillet from heat. Spoon marinara sauce over and around cutlets. Sprinkle 1 teaspoon mozzarella over each cutlet, and then sprinkle 2 teaspoons parmesan over each. Sprinkle butter pieces atop the cutlets. Bake until cheese melts and chicken is cooked through, about 3–5 minutes. Serve over angel hair pasta.

Simple Marinara Sauce

½ cup extra-virgin olive oil
1 small onion, chopped
2 cloves garlic, chopped
1 stalk celery, chopped
1 carrot, chopped
salt and pepper to taste
2 can crushed tomatoes
4-6 basil leaves
2 dry bay leaves
4 Tbsp. butter

In a large pot, heat oil over medium heat. Add onion and garlic and sauté until soft and translucent, about 2 minutes. Add celery and carrots and season with salt and pepper. Sauté until all the vegetables are soft, about 5 minutes. Add tomatoes, basil, and bay leaves and simmer covered on low heat for 1 hour or until thick. Remove bay leaves. Add butter. Add half the tomato sauce into the bowl of a food processor. Process until smooth. Continue with remaining tomato sauce. If not using all the sauce, allow it to cool completely and pour 1 to 2 cup portions into freezer plastic bags. This will freeze up to 6 months.

pasta with shrimp, Asparagus, and Tomatoes

4 oz. dried spaghetti
12 oz. frozen shrimp
16 thin spears fresh asparagus
1 tsp. olive oil
4 cloves garlic, minced
2 cups Roma tomatoes
¼ cup chicken broth
chopped
¼ tsp. ground pepper
1 Tbsp. butter
¼ cup fresh basil

Cook pasta according to package directions. Drain; keep warm. Meanwhile, thaw shrimp if frozen. Set aside. Snap off and discard woody bases from asparagus. Remove tips; set aside. Cut asparagus diagonally into 1 inch pieces; set aside. In a medium sauce pan, heat olive oil, adding minced garlic, asparagus, and Roma tomatoes. Cook 4 minutes. Add broth, butter, pepper, and fresh basil. Add the shrimp at the end, and ladle onto the hot pasta. Serve with garlic bread.

pesto pizza
and Artichokes

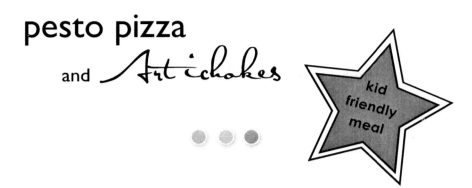

Make pizza crust as explained in the recipe for Barbecue Chicken Pizza. To make pesto:

½ cup packed fresh basil
¼ cup fresh parsley
¼ cup fresh grated parmesan
2 Tbsp. pine nuts
1 large garlic clove
2 Tbsp. olive oil
2 Tbsp. butter, softened
¼ tsp. salt
fresh pepper

Place all ingredients in a food processor, and blend until smooth. For leftovers, simply pour the pesto into ice cube trays in the freezer, and then transfer to a freezer bag when frozen. This way you can have fresh pesto whenever you desire!

To make pizza

Spread a thin layer of pesto over the uncooked pizza rounds. Top with artichokes, diced tomatoes, and more parmesan cheese. Shredded chicken is optional. Bake on medium low on the bbq or in the oven until cheese melts, and dough is lightly golden.

Kid-Friendly Recipe: Instead of pesto sauce, use spaghetti sauce, and substitute pepperoni and mozzarella for the other toppings.

chicken lasagna rolls
with Chive Cream Sauce

6 dried lasagna noodles
8 oz. cream cheese, softened
½ cup milk
¼ cup grated parmesan
1 Tbsp. snipped fresh chives
1 cup purchased pasta sauce
1½ cups chopped, cooked chicken
⅛ tsp. ground pepper
½ cup bottled roasted red sweet peppers, drained, sliced
1 cup frozen broccoli, drained

Preheat oven to 350 degrees. Cook noodles according to package directions. Drain noodles; rinse with cold water. Drain again. Cut each in half crosswise; set aside. Meanwhile in a bowl, beat cream cheese with an electric mixer on medium to high speed for 30 seconds. Slowly beat in milk. Stir in cheese and chives. In a bowl, combine ½ cup white sauce, chicken, broccoli, roasted peppers, and black pepper. Place about ¼ cup filling at one end of each noodle. Roll up. Place rolls, seam sides down, in a 3-qt. baking dish. Spoon marinara sauce over rolls. Spoon remaining white sauce over top. Cover and bake for 35–40 minutes or until heated through.

ASIAN

Sweet and Sour Chicken 106
Asian Beef and Noodle Bowl .. 107
Curry in a Hurry 108
Ginger Chicken Stir Fry 109
Sweet and Spicy Sesame
    Noodles and Jerk Chicken .. 110
Teriyaki Salmon 111

sweet and sour chicken
with Rice

4 large chicken breasts
1 egg, beaten
½ cup cornstarch
1 tsp. garlic salt
4 Tbsp. oil

Cut each chicken breast into 2-inch cubes or into strips. Dip each piece first into the beaten egg, and then dredge it in the cornstarch mixed with garlic salt. Place chicken pieces into a skillet with 4 Tbsp. oil, and brown on both sides until nicely golden. Transfer chicken to a baking dish; do not overlap the chicken. Pour the sweet and sour sauce over the top. Bake at 350 degrees for 30 minutes. Serve over rice and a side of steamed green beans.

Sweet & Sour Sauce

¾ cups sugar
¼ cup pineapple juice
1 Tbsp. soy sauce
½ cup red wine vinegar
3 Tbsp. ketchup
1 tsp. salt

Combine all ingredients in a small saucepan and simmer until smooth.

asian beef and Noodle Bowl

4 cups water
2 pkgs. ramen noodles (any flavor)
2 tsp. oil plus a kick of cayenne
12 oz. thin beef flank
1 tsp. grated fresh ginger
2 cloves garlic, minced
1 cup beef broth
2 Tbsp. soy sauce
2 cups baby spinach, torn
1 cup shredded carrots
¼ cup shipped fresh cilantro

In a large saucepan, bring water to boiling. If desired, break up noodles; drop noodles into boiling water.

Discard flavor packets. Return to boiling for 3 minutes. Drain noodles; set aside. Meanwhile, in a very large skillet, heat oil over medium high heat. Add beef, ginger, and garlic; cook and stir for 2–3 minutes or until beef is desired doneness. Carefully stir beef broth and soy sauce into skillet; stir to combine. Heat through. Stir in cilantro just before serving.

curry in a hurry

4 chicken breasts
¼ cup flour
¼ cup butter
½ cup chopped onion
¼ cup celery, sliced thinly
¼ cup golden raisins
¾ cups chicken broth
1 cup half and half or milk
2 Tbsp. curry
salt and pepper to taste

Boil chicken and cut into chunks. Put aside. Melt butter, and sauté onion, celery, and raisins until tender. Add chicken broth and milk. Cook uncovered 5 minutes. Stir in curry, salt and pepper, and 2 teaspoons Garam Marsala if desired. Simmer 10 minutes. Add chicken, and serve over steamed rice. This dish is also delicious with a side of steamed, buttered sliced carrots and a touch of brown sugar.

ginger chicken stir fry

1 Tbsp. cooking oil or peanut oil
1 medium zucchini, sliced thin
1 medium carrot, sliced thin
1 small onion, sliced thin
1 small red sweet pepper, halved and sliced thin
½ head small green cabbage, shred
12 oz. chicken, cut into 1-inch pieces
½ cup bottled stir fry sauce
½ tsp. ground ginger
hot cooked rice
peanuts, cashews, or toasted sliced almonds (optional)

Heat oil in a wok or skillet. Add cubed chicken and allow to cook until browned. Add all other ingredients, and cook just until tender-crisp. Serve over hot cooked rice, and top with nuts, if desired.

sweet and spicy sesame noodles and Jerk Chicken

*YUM!
Rick says "tastes like Yakisoba"*

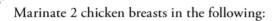

kid friendly meal

Marinate 2 chicken breasts in the following:

juice of 2 limes
½ cup orange juice
1 tsp. each paprika, cumin, allspice
¼ tsp. cinnamon
1 tsp. thyme
½ cup olive oil
½ tsp. salt

When chicken is done, sauté until tender and ready to shred.

1 lb. spaghetti
½ cup chicken stock
1 tsp. fresh ginger
1 clove garlic, grated
3 Tbsp. peanut butter
¼ cup soy sauce
2 Tbsp. oil
2 Tbsp. honey
1 red pepper, sliced thin
green onions
pineapple chunks

Cook pasta. Heat chicken stock in a small saucepan. Add ginger, garlic, peanut butter, soy sauce, canola oil, and honey and whisk to combine. In a large bowl combine pasta and sauce. Sprinkle with onions and sesame seeds.

Kid-Friendly Recipe: Instead of shredding the chicken, brown the chicken chunks and serve them on a skewer. Offer a dipping sauce of 1 Tbsp. honey and ½ tsp. Dijon mustard on the side. Serve with pineapple chunks, if desired.

teriyaki salmon

This recipe is mouth-wateringly delicious, but remember to allow yourself a few extra hours so the salmon can marinate!

1 lb. salmon, skin removed
5 garlic cloves, slivered
1 (1-inch) piece gingerroot, slivered
juice of 1 lemon
¼ cup teriyaki marinade
2 Tbsp. frozen orange juice concentrate

Make slits on both sides of the salmon. Insert the garlic slivers, alternately with the ginger root slivers. Drench both sides of the salmon with lemon juice. Place in an ungreased baking dish. Pour teriyaki sauce over the salmon. Spoon the unthawed orange juice concentrate over the salmon. Marinate the salmon in the refrigerator for 1 to 2 hours. Turn the salmon once and let marinate for an additional 1 hour. Preheat the oven to 350 degrees. Remove the salmon from the refrigerator so that the salmon and baking dish can both warm up before baking. Discard the marinade. Bake for 20 to 30 minutes or until the salmon flakes easily with a fork. Be careful not to overcook.

MEXICAN/ SOUTHWESTERN

Southwestern Egg Rolls 114
Chicken Fajitas 115
Navajo Tacos 116
Black Beans and Spanish Rice .. 118
Creamy Chicken Enchiladas 119
Turkey Chili 120
White Lightning Chili 122

southwestern egg rolls

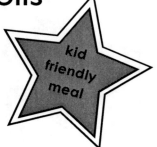

2 chicken breasts, diced
½ red pepper, minced
2 Tbsp. green onion, minced
¼ cup white onion, minced
1 can corn
1 can black beans, drained
2 Tbsp. spinach, sliced thinly
1 small can green chilies
½ tsp. chili powder
½ tsp. cumin
½ Tbsp. fresh parsley, minced
¼ tsp. salt
1 cup jack or cheddar cheese, shredded
flour tortillas

Avocado-ranch dipping sauce

1 cup ranch dressing
1 avocado, mashed
1 tsp. onion, minced
salt and pepper to taste
1 Tbsp. lime juice

Cook chicken and dice. In a large bowl, mix all egg roll ingredients together, except flour tortillas and cheese. Saute all ingredients until warm. Remove from heat and add shredded cheese. Mix well. Warm tortillas. Place 1 cup of mixture inside each tortilla. Fold completely together so mixture can not escape. Place inside a panini grill and melt cheese. Serve with dipping sauce. To make dipping sauce, simply combine all ingredients in a food processor until smooth.

Kid-Friendly Recipe: Lay out each tortilla and top with diced chicken and shredded cheese. Fold the tortilla in half, and grill on the panini press. Serve along side a fresh salad of spinach, red pepper slices, and corn.

chicken fajitas

3 chicken breasts
1 small onion, thinly sliced
multi-color peppers, sliced thin
½ cup salsa
1 tsp. cumin or taco seasoning
½ tsp. garlic powder
steak and shrimp, optional

Cook chicken in small amount of olive oil until browned. Season with garlic and taco seasoning. Remove from heat, and cook remaining ingredients. Serve with tortillas, lettuce, salsa, tomatoes, cheese, sour cream, guacamole, and so forth.

navajo tacos

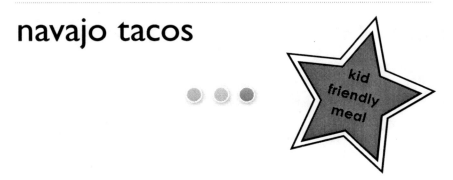

I like to serve this with buttermilk scones, then layer all the toppings on top!

Buttermilk Scones

    1 quart buttermilk, warm
    2 eggs
    2 Tbsp. oil
    2 Tbsp. yeast
    2 Tbsp. sugar
    1½ tsp. salt
    1 Tbsp. baking powder
    ½ tsp. baking soda
    6–8 cups flour

Combine all ingredients in a large mixing bowl. Knead 6 minutes until dough is soft, but still sticky. Allow to rise 1 hour. With a floured hand, tear off small handfuls of dough, and stretch out thinly into discs. Allow to rise a little on the countertop while you preheat the oil. You'll know the oil is hot enough if you put in your scone dough and it immediately floats to the top. Brown on both sides, and then place on a paper towel until ready to serve. Top with all the toppings below:

Kid-Friendly Recipe: Simply serve the Navajo tacos with honey butter and fresh fruit on the side or a small bowl of chili (below) sprinkled with cheddar cheese.

Navajo Taco Toppings

I like to make my own chili sauce to go on top of the tacos, but if you're pressed for time, you can simply open a can of chili and then add the other toppings.

- 1 lb. ground beef
- ½ onion, chopped
- 3 Tbsp. ketchup
- 1 can tomato sauce
- 1 tsp. mustard
- 1 tsp. brown sugar
- 1 tsp. Worcestershire sauce
- ¼ tsp. salt
- 1 pkg. taco seasoning
- ¼ cup or more water

Brown ground beef and onion in a skillet and drain. Add the rest of the ingredients and simmer until thick, adding more water for a runnier consistency. Place a small ladleful of sauce over warm scones, and then add the following toppings:

- cheddar cheese, grated
- iceberg lettuce, chopped
- olives, sliced
- tomatoes, sliced
- guacamole
- sour cream

black beans and Spanish Rice

Spanish Rice Blend

    4 cups uncooked long grain rice
    2 tsp. cumin
    1 Tbsp. chili powder
    1 tsp. salt

Combine all ingredients, and place in a storage container. To make 4 servings of rice, simply combine 1 cup of rice blend with 2 ½ cups of water and 2 Tbsp. butter, and cook just as you would regular rice.

Black Bean Topping

    2 Tbsp. oil
    ½ lb. lean ground beef
    1 cup onion, chopped
    1 can green chilies
    1 clove garlic, minced

Saute all these ingredients together, and set aside. Meanwhile, in a bowl, combine the following:

    1 Tbsp. lemon juice
    1 Tbsp. mustard
    1 tsp. chili powder
    2 Tbsp. soy sauce
    dash of cayenne pepper
    1 cup tomato sauce

Combine all these ingredients to the meat mixture and simmer 20 minutes on low. Add 2 cups black beans that have been cooked and drained. Serve over warm Spanish rice, and garnish with shredded lettuce, a little shredded cheese, and a dollop of sour cream.

creamy chicken enchiladas

OK. needs more spice

1 can cream of chicken soup
1 onion, chopped
½ cup sour cream
1 tsp. chili powder
1 Tbsp. butter
2 cups chopped chicken
1 small can green chilies
1 cup cheddar, grated
8 small tortillas

Preheat oven to 350. In a small bowl, mix the soup and sour cream. Melt butter over medium heat. Add onion and chili powder and sauté until tender. Stir in the chicken, green chilies, and 2 tablespoons soup mix. Cook until heated through. Spread ½ cup of soup mix in a 9x13 baking dish. Spoon about ¼ cup of chicken in the center of each tortilla. Roll them up, seam side down, and spoon remaining soup mixture on top. Sprinkle with cheese. Bake 25 minutes until bubbly.

turkey chili and Cornbread Muffins

2 lbs. lean ground turkey
1 Tbsp. apple cider vinegar
1 large onion, chopped
3 Tbsp. brown sugar
2 Tbsp. chopped dehydrated peppers
1 Tbsp. mustard
3 cups water
1 cup ketchup
1 Tbsp. chili powder
1 Tbsp. paprika
1 Tbsp. sea salt
1 can corn with juice
2 cans diced tomatoes with juice
2 cans kidney beans, drained

In your electric pressure cooker, brown the turkey, along with the onion and green peppers until cooked through. Add all the remaining ingredients and cover with the lid. Cook on high for 15 minutes. Serve with cornbread muffins.

Cornbread Muffins

1½ cups fine yellow cornmeal*
1²/₃ cups all purpose flour
½ cup sugar
2 Tbsp. baking powder
1 tsp. salt
1²/₃ cups whole milk
4 large eggs, lightly beaten
½ cup plus 2½ Tbsp. butter

Preheat the oven to 375. Lightly grease or line a muffin pan. In a large bowl, stir together the cornmeal, flour, sugar, baking powder, and salt. Make a well and pour in the milk, eggs, and melted butter. Stir together the wet and dry ingredients just until combined. Take care not to over-mix; the batter should be slightly lumpy. Pour batter into the prepared muffin pan. Bake until the muffins are golden brown around the edges and on top (25–30 minutes). Let stand 15 minutes, and serve while warm.

*To grind your own fresh cornmeal, place 1 cup popcorn kernels in your electric grinder on coarse setting. Store the leftovers in a container in the fridge.

white lightning chili and

- 1 lb. Great Northern Beans, cooked, drained
- 6 cups chicken broth
- 2 garlic cloves
- 1 Tbsp. cumin
- 2 tsp. oregano
- 2 cans green chilies
- 2 medium onions, chopped
- 3 cups chicken, cooked, cube
- 2 Tbsp. oil
- 1 cup sour cream,
- jack cheese

In a large stock pot, sauté chilies, garlic, and onions in 2 Tbsp. oil until tender. Add all other ingredients except sour cream and cheese. Cook 40 minutes on low, and just before serving, stir in 1 cup sour cream and sprinkle with shredded jack cheese.

Cornbread

- 2 cups biscuit mix
- 1 cup milk
- 1/3 cup cornmeal
- ¾ cups oil
- ½ tsp. baking soda
- 2 eggs
- 1 cup sugar

Combine all ingredients and bake at 350 in an 8x8 pan for 25–30 minutes, until golden.

VEGETARIAN

Lasagna of Roasted
    Butternut Squash 124
Potato Latkes with Sour Cream
    and Applesauce 125
Eggplant Roll-ups 126
Stuffed Zucchini Quinoa 127
Roasted Sweet Potato
    and Apple Soup 128

lasagna of roasted
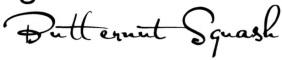

3 lbs. butternut squash, quartered, peeled, and diced
3 Tbsp. olive oil
salt and pepper to taste
4 cups milk
2 Tbsp. dried rosemary, crumbled
1 Tbsp. minced garlic
¼ cup butter
1 cup flour
9 sheets dry lasagna noodles
1⅓ cups parmesan, grated
1 cup heavy whipping cream
½ tsp. salt

Preheat the oven to 450 degrees. Oil 2 large-rimmed baking sheets. Toss squash and olive oil together to coat the squash. Spread squash in a single layer on the baking sheets and place in the oven, baking 10 minutes. Season with salt, and bake 15 minutes longer; then remove from oven.

Mix the milk and rosemary in a saucepan and simmer 10 minutes. Strain the mixture through a fine sieve into a pitcher. Cook the garlic and butter until softened. Stir in the flour, and cook 3 minutes, stirring constantly. Remove from heat, and whisk in the milk mixture in a slow stream until smooth. Return the skillet to the heat and simmer the sauce 10 minutes, stirring occasionally.

Add the cooked squash, salt, and pepper. Reduce oven heat to 375, and grease a 9x13 baking pan. Beat cream and salt in a bowl with an electric mixer until it holds soft peaks. Layer 1 cup of the sauce, ⅓ of the lasagna sheets, ½ of the remaining sauce, ½ cup of the cheese, ⅓ of the lasagna sheets, the remaining sauce, ½ cup of the cheese, the remaining lasagna sheets, all the cream mixture, and the remaining cheese in the baking dish. Cover the baking dish with foil, tenting if necessary so the foil does not touch the cream layer. Bake 35 minutes. Remove the foil and bake for 15 minutes longer, until the lasagna is bubbling and golden brown. Let stand for 5 minutes before serving.

potato latkes with sour cream and *Applesauce*

1½ cups dehydrated shredded potatoes
2 eggs
¼ cup grated onion
1 tsp. salt
½ tsp. ground pepper
⅓ cup frying oil
applesauce
sour cream

Place shredded potatoes in a medium bowl, and cover with boiling water. After 30 minutes, drain water, squeezing as much excess water out as possible. In a smaller bowl, combine grated onion, eggs, salt, and pepper. Add to potatoes and set aside. In a frying pan, place oil, and allow to heat until ready to fry. Drop potato mixture into pan by ¼ cup-full, and flatten slightly. Brown for several minutes, on each side until golden and crispy. Drain on paper towels. While still hot, serve with a dollop of sour cream and a dollop of applesauce. Serve with a side of sausage links for a dinnertime breakfast.

eggplant roll-ups

1 large eggplant, cut lengthwise into ¼ inch strips
canola oil spray
16 oz. ricotta cheese
1 tsp. basil
¼ cup grated parmesan cheese
½ tsp. salt
⅛ tsp. pepper

Sauce

½ cup chopped onion
3 cloves minced garlic
½ tsp. thyme
2 Tbsp. olive oil
16 oz. can diced tomato
salt and pepper to taste

Preheat broiler. Place foil in the bottom of a broiler pan. Place eggplant in pan and spray with canola oil. Broil until light brown. Turn the eggplant and repeat.

Reduce oven temperature to 400 degrees. Grease a 7x11 inch baking pan. Mix ricotta cheese, basil, parmesan cheese, salt, and pepper in a bowl. Place a scoop of the cheese mixture on 1 end of each eggplant strip. Roll strip around the cheese mixture and place seam side down in the pan.

For the sauce: Saute the onion, garlic, and thyme in the olive oil in a saucepan until soft. Add tomatoes, salt, and pepper, and simmer 5 to 10 minutes. Spoon sauce over rolls. Bake 20 to 30 minutes.

stuffed zucchini and quinoa

½ cup white quinoa, rinsed
4 medium zucchini
1 can cannelloni beans
1 cup grape tomatoes
½ cup almonds, chopped
2 cloves garlic, minced
¾ cups grated parmesan
4 Tbsp. olive oil

Heat oven to 400 degrees. In a large skillet, combine quinoa and 1 cup water and bring to a boil. Reduce heat to medium low, cover, and simmer until it's tender and water is absorbed, about 12 minutes. Meanwhile, cut zucchini in half lengthwise and scoop out seeds. Arrange in a large baking dish, cut-side up. Fluff quinoa and fold in beans, tomatoes, almonds, garlic, ½ cup parmesan, and 3 tablespoons oil. Spoon mixture into zucchini. Top with remaining tablespoon of oil and ¼ cup parmesan. Cover with foil and bake until zucchini is tender, 25–30 minutes. Remove foil and bake until golden, 8–10 minutes.

roasted sweet potato and apple soup

with *Cucumber Goat Cheese Sandwiches*

kid friendly meal

These sandwiches are really the best companion to this delicious fall-time soup!

Soup

    3 lbs. sweet potatoes
    1 Tbsp. olive oil
    1 onion, chopped
    1 celery stalk, sliced
    1 granny smith apple, thinly sliced

Heat oven to 400 degrees. Prick the potatoes with a fork, placing them on a baking sheet, and roast until tender, 40–45 minutes. Meanwhile, heat the oil in a large saucepan over medium high heat. Add the onion, celery, and apple and cook, stirring occasionally, until soft, 10–12 minutes. Halve the potatoes, scooping out the flesh, and add to the saucepan. Add 6 cups water, 2 tsp. salt, and ½ tsp. pepper. Cook until heated through, 8–10 minutes. Puree the soup in the blender. Add water if necessary to reach the desired consistency.

Sandwiches

    16 slices whole-grain bread
    2 4-oz. logs fresh goat cheese
    1 cup walnuts, chopped
    2 cucumbers, thinly sliced
    1 bunch watercress, stems removed

Spread 8 slices of bread with goat cheese. Top with walnuts, cucumbers, watercress, and the remaining 8 slices of bread.

Kid-Friendly Recipe: Spread the bread with a thin layer of cream cheese. Then top with thinly sliced cucumbers and apples. Try serving up the soup in mini pumpkins to add some pizzazz!

TRADITIONAL ENTREES

Italian Crock-pot Chicken 130
Mediterranean Lentil Burgers .. 131
Coconut Salmon 132
Salisbury Steak 133
Creamy Coleslaw and
    Halibut 134
Chicken and Broccoli 135
Fetuccini Chicken and Bean 136
Stuffed Cabbage Rolls 137
Tender Roast and
    Red Cabbage 138
Baked Salmon with Spinach
    and Mushrooms 139

Chicken Cordon Bleu 140
Oven Roasted Salmon with
    Spinach and Coconut 142
Toasty, Cozy Shepherd's Pie 143
Porcupine Meatballs with
    Rice 144
Stuffed Green Peppers 145
Italian Braided Meat Loaf 146
Chicken Florentine 148
Grilled Lemon Chicken and
    Coconut Rice 149
Ultimate Shrimp Scampi 150

italian crock-pot chicken

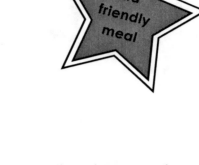

4 chicken breasts
1 can cream of chicken soup
1 (8-oz.) pkg. cream cheese
1 can cream of mushroom soup
1 pkg. Italian dressing mix
1 cup milk

Place the 4 chicken breasts in a Crock-Pot. Combine the soups and softened cream cheese, adding the Italian dressing mix and the milk. Stir until well combined, and pour over the chicken breasts. Turn the Crock-Pot on low, and allow to cook until bubbly, and the chicken is tender and easily shredded, about 6 hours. Serve over rice or pasta.

Kid-Friendly Recipe

4 flour tortillas
¼ cup cream cheese, softened
1 tomato, chopped
Shredded cooked chicken 4 leaves Romaine lettuce
Ranch dip, optional

Spread each tortilla with ½ Tbsp. cream cheese. Top with shredded chicken, tomatoes, and 1 leaf of lettuce. Roll up tightly, and serve as a roll-up. Dip in ranch dressing if desired.

mediterranean lentil burgers
with Cucumber Sauce

kid friendly meal

- 1 lb. ground turkey
- ¼ cup lentils, cooked
- ½ small onion, peeled and grated
- ¼ cup bread crumb
- 1 egg, lightly beaten
- 1 tsp. curry
- 1 tsp. salt
- ½ tsp. pepper
- juice of 1 large lime
- cucumber yogurt sauce (below)
- chopped tomatoes
- shredded lettuce
- whole pita

Combine turkey, lentils, onion, bread crumbs, egg, curry, salt, pepper, and lime juice in a mixing bowl. Mix with clean hands or a wooden spoon. Form meat into 8 small patties shaped like flattened ovals. Cook on a hot grill or broil in the oven 5 to 8 minutes on each side, until cooked through. Serve with Cucumber Yogurt Sauce, chopped tomatoes, and shredded lettuce in pita.

Cucumber Yogurt Sauce
- 1 small cucumber, peeled and minced
- 2 cups plain yogurt
- ½ tsp. sea salt
- 2 tsp. dried mint
- ½ tsp. sugar

Combine all ingredients, and refrigerate until ready to use. Pour into pita over the patties and other fillings. Makes 2 cups.

Kid-Friendly Recipe: Instead of forming the meat mixture into patties, simply brown the meat similar to making tacos. Spoon ¼ cup meat mixture into the pita, and then top with shredded cheese. Serve with tomato wedges and cucumber yogurt dip on the side.

coconut salmon

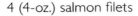
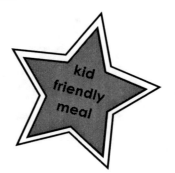

4 (4-oz.) salmon filets
2 cups orange juice
1 egg, beaten
1 (7-oz.) pkg. flaked coconut
4 Tbsp. orange marmalade
1 Tbsp. Dijon mustard.

Place filets in a medium bowl with orange juice, and marinade 8 hours or overnight in the refrigerator. Preheat oven to 350. Coat salmon fillets with egg, and then dredge in coconut. Arrange in a single layer in a baking dish. Bake 15 minutes, until coconut is golden brown and the fish is easily flaked with a fork. In a small pan, blend orange marmalade and Dijon mustard over medium heat until warm. Serve as a dipping sauce for the salmon. Serve with steamed broccoli

Kid-Friendly Recipe: Without marinading the salmon, place the salmon on the same baking dish, sprinkled with lemon pepper, and bake along with the marinated salmon until lightly golden. Serve with fresh orange wedges and steamed broccoli.

salisbury steak
with Mashed Potatoes

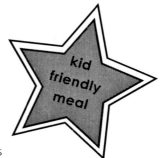

2 cans cream of mushroom soup
1 egg, beaten
1 lb. ground beef
¼ cup chopped onion
⅓ cup dry bread crumbs or ground oats
1½ cups mushrooms, sliced

In a bowl, combine ¼ cup soup, ground beef, bread crumbs, egg, and onion. Shape into 6 patties. Cook over medium heat in a skillet until browned on both sides. Stir together soup and a little milk. Pour mixture over beef patties, and cover the skillet with a lid, reducing heat to a simmer for 20 minutes. Serve over mashed potatoes.

Kid-Friendly Recipe: To make hamburger patties, combine ½ lb. meat with 2 Tbsp. ground oats or bread crumbs. Add seasoning of your choice. Brown patties, and serve in a whole wheat bun. Serve with fresh fruit.

creamy coleslaw
and Halibut

½ onion, chopped
½ tsp. salt
½ cup sugar
¼ tsp. ground pepper
½ cup vegetable oil
1 cabbage, shredded
¼ cup cider vinegar
3 Tbsp. mayonnaise
¼ tsp. celery seeds

Combine onion and sugar in a bowl. Cover and let stand 30 minutes. Pour onion mixture into a blender. Add oil, vinegar, mayonnaise, celery seeks, salt, and pepper. Blend well. Cover and refrigerate for at least 1 hour. Just before serving, toss dressing with cabbage.

Halibut

In a lightly oiled pan, place 4 halibut fillets. Sprinkle with lemon pepper and brown each side until golden. Sprinkle generously with fresh lemon juice. Serve with coleslaw.

chicken and broccoli

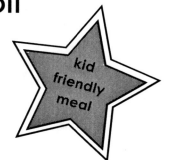

4 breasts of chicken, cooked and diced
4 cups broccoli, steamed
1 can cream of chicken soup
½ cup mayonnaise
½ cup milk
2 tsp. lemon juice
1 cup shredded cheddar cheese
buttered cracker crumbs

In an 8x8 inch baking dish, place the chopped steamed broccoli. Layer with the cubed chicken. Combine the soup, mayonnaise, milk, lemon juice, and shredded cheddar cheese. Then pour over chicken and broccoli. Sprinkle generously with buttered cracker crumbs. Cover with foil, and then bake in a preheated 350 degree oven for 40 minutes until cooked and bubbly. Serve over hot rice.

Kid-Friendly Recipe: Instead of cooking the chicken, cut the breasts into long strips. Dredge in a little milk, and then dip into a mixture of ¼ cup flour and 2 tsp. lemon pepper. Saute in some olive oil until golden brown. Serve with hot buttered rice and steamed broccoli topped with shredded cheese.

fetuccini chicken and bean

8 oz. fetuccini
2 chicken breasts, cubed.
3 Tbsp. butter, divided
¼ cup chopped green onion
2 tsp. garlic, minced
¼ cup flour
1 tsp. basil
2 cups milk
1 can red beans
½ cup frozen peas
½ cup grated parmesan cheese

Cook pasta. Saute chicken in 1 tablespoons butter until browned. Remove. Add green onions, and garlic, and sauté in 2 tablespoons butter. Stir in flour, basil, and cook for 2 minutes. Add milk, and boil until thickened. Stir in chicken beans, peas. Cook 5 minutes. Add cheese until melted. Serve over fetuccini.

stuffed cabbage rolls

1 cup cooked rice
1 egg, slightly beaten
1 tsp. salt
¼ tsp. pepper
8 cabbage leaves
1 lb. lean ground beef
1 can tomato soup
¼ cup chopped onion

Bring a large pan of lightly salted water to a boil. Add cabbage leaves and cook for 2–4 minutes, or until softened. Drain. In a medium mixing bowl, combine ground beef, 1 cup rice, onion, 1 egg, salt, pepper, and 2 tablespoons tomato soup. Mix thoroughly. Divide beef mixture evenly among cabbage leaves. Roll and secure with toothpicks. In a large skillet over medium heat, place the cabbage rolls, and pour the remaining soup over the top. Cover and bring to a boil, then reduce heat to a simmer for 40 minutes, stirring and basting with the liquid until done.

tender roast and Red Cabbage

1 (3–4 lb.) roast of choice
onion soup mix*

2 Tbsp. oil
pepper

Rub roast with a generous helping of pepper. In a deep skillet, brown roast in 2 Tbsp. hot oil, turning to brown all sides. Transfer roast into a Crock-Pot, and cover with onion soup mix. Add 1 cup water, and turn the Crock-Pot to high for 2 hours. Then reduce to low for 4 more hours or until tender and falling apart.

*To make your own onion soup mix, combine the following ingredients, and store in an airtight container until ready to use. Use in any recipe that calls for own onion soup mix.

- 1/3 cup dehydrated chopped onions
- ½ cup beef bouillon soup base
- ½ cup dehydrated butter
- 2 Tbsp. cornstarch
- 2 tsp. onion powder
- 2 tsp. parsley flakes (optional)

Red Cabbage

1 large head red cabbage
2 Tbsp. butter
2 cups vinegar

1 cup water
1½ cups sugar

Boil all ingredients together in a large saucepan for 2 minutes. Then place the lid on the pan, and simmer for 3 hours. Remove the lid and simmer 1 more hour. Serve along side the tender roast. Also delicious with mashed potatoes and gravy!

baked salmon
with Spinach and Mushrooms

4 salmon fillets
2 cups chopped fresh spinach
1 cup sliced mushrooms
1 medium tomato, chopped
1/3 cup sun dried tomato vinaigrette (Kraft)

Place salmon filets, skin sides down, in a 13x9 inch dish, sprayed with cooking spray. Mix remaining ingredients until well blended; spoon over salmon. Serve with a baked potato.

chicken cordon blue and *Rice Pilaf*

6 chicken breasts, boneless, skinless
½ lb. sliced Swiss cheese
¼ lb. sliced ham
1 stick melted butter
1 cup cracker crumbs

Cut chicken breasts in half. Pound and flatten them with a rolling pin or meat tenderizer between 2 layers of wax paper. Place a slice of cheese on each breast, followed by a slice of ham. Lightly salt and pepper the ham, then roll up in a bundle, and secure with toothpicks if necessary. Dip each bundle in the melted butter, and then cover with cracker crumbs. Bake in a 325 degree oven in a baking dish for 40 minutes. Before serving, drizzle with sauce, below:

Sauce

1 can cream of mushroom soup cup sour cream
2 tsp. lemon juice
2 Tbsp. milk

Combine all ingredients in a small saucepan and heat until bubbly. Serve over chicken.

Rice Pilaf

4 Tbsp. butter
1 cup spaghetti, broken in ½ inches
1½ cups long grain rice
¼ tsp. salt

1 tsp. pepper
5 cups chicken broth
2 tsp. parsley

Melt butter over medium heat in a saucepan. Stir in pasta and rice until golden brown. Slowly add chicken broth to rice mixture. Turn to high heat until rice comes to boil. Cover and simmer 20 minutes or until rice is fluffy. Add the parsley, and cover again, turning off the heat and allowing the rice to rest 10 minutes before serving.

oven roasted salmon
with Spinach and Coconut

1 Tbsp. olive oil
2 lbs. salmon fillets
½ tsp. seasoned salt
1 bag baby spinach
¼ cup heavy whipping cream
3 Tbsp. flaked, sweetened coconut

Place rack in the center of the oven, and preheat the oven to 400 degrees. Pour olive oil into a large ovenproof skillet and heat it over medium-high heat. Season the salmon with salt on both sides. When the olive oil is hot, add the salmon and cook it until lightly browned, 1–2 minutes. Remove salmon from the skillet and set aside. Add spinach to the pan juices in the skillet. Pour cream over the spinach and sprinkle the coconut on top. Place salmon pieces back in the skillet on top of spinach and place skillet in the oven. Bake salmon until it is opaque and the juices are bubbling, 7–8 minutes. Serve at once. Tastes great with garlic mashed potatoes.

toasty, cozy shepherd's pie

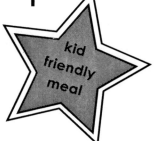

1 lb. stew meat or meatballs
oil for browning
1 clove garlic, minced
1½ cups beef broth
½ tsp. each Cajun seasoning and dried basil
¼ tsp. each dried thyme and pepper
4 cups frozen mixed vegetables
1 cup onion, chopped
½ cup water
1 Tbsp. brown gravy mix
2 lbs. mashed potatoes
1 Tbsp. chives, chopped
½ cup mozzarella cheese

Brown stew meat over medium high heat. Add garlic and sauté 20 seconds. Add broth, and spices to meat and simmer covered for 30 minutes. Simmer vegetables in 3 cups of water until tender. Mix ½ cup water and gravy mix in a bowl. Add to mixture, and simmer 5 minutes. Mix chives with mashed potatoes. Place the meat mixture in the bottom of a 2½-quart casserole dish. Top with mashed potatoes. Sprinkle with cheese, and bake at 375 for 12 minutes.

Kid-Friendly Recipe: Bake meatballs in a 350 degree oven for 25 minutes or until golden brown. Serve with mashed potatoes and a small portion of steamed mixed vegetables.

porcupine meatballs with rice

1½ lbs. lean ground beef
²/₃ cups raw long grain rice
½ cup water
¼ cup finely chopped onion
1 tsp. seasoned salt
¼ tsp. garlic powder
⅛ tsp. pepper
1 large can tomato sauce
1 cup water
2 tsp. Worcestershire sauce

Mix ground beef with the rice, ½ cup water, onion, salt, garlic powder, and pepper. Shape into 1½-inch balls. Place meatballs in an ungreased 2-quart shallow baking dish. Mix the remaining ingredients and pour over porcupine meatballs. Cover with foil, and bake at 350 degrees for 45 minutes. Uncover and bake an additional 20 minutes.

stuffed green peppers

4 medium green bell peppers
1 lb. lean ground beef
¼ cup finely chopped onion
1½ cups cooked rice
1 tsp. seasoned salt
½ tsp. black pepper
1 large jar spaghetti sauce

In a bowl, mix the onion, ground beef, rice, salt, and pepper. Cut tops off green peppers, and remove any seeds. Stuff each pepper with equal amounts of meat mixture. Place peppers in the Crock-Pot, and cover with spaghetti sauce. Allow to cook 6 hours on low, or just until peppers are tender.

italian braided meat loaf

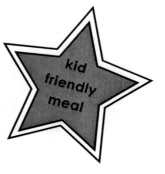

kid friendly meal

This is a great way to use your dehydrated vegetables such as onions, peppers, and mushrooms. If you're using fresh vegetables, you'll use 3 times the amount given for dry.

Bread Shell

1 tsp. SAF yeast
2 Tbsp. cornmeal
½ cups warm water
Italian Herb Filling (see below)
2 tsp. sugar
1 cup grated mozzarella cheese
1 tsp. salt
¼ cup grated parmesan cheese
2 cups flour
water
1 Tbsp. vegetable oil
sesame seeds

Italian Herb Filling

1 lb. lean ground beef
¼ tsp. basil
1 Tbsp. flour
1 tsp. paprika
2 Tbsp. onion flakes
⅓ tsp. salt
2 Tbsp. dried chopped green pepper
⅓ cup pitted black olives, chopped
3 Tbsp. dried mushrooms or 1 (4-oz.) can mushrooms
1 Tbsp. Worcestershire sauce
1 (8-oz.) can tomato sauce

1 fresh garlic clove, crushed
1 cup water
½ tsp. oregano

In a medium bowl, dissolve yeast in warm water. Add sugar, salt, and 1–1½ cups flour. Beat until smooth. Gradually add enough remaining flour to make a stiff dough. Turn out onto a floured surface and begin kneading, adding only enough flour to prevent dough from sticking to surface. Knead until satiny, 5–10 minutes. Coat the inside of a large bowl with 1 Tbsp. oil. Place dough in bowl, turning once.

Cover with a cloth. Set in a warm place free from drafts and let rise until doubled in bulk, about 1 hour. Preheat oven to 400 degrees. Sprinkle a jelly-roll pan or large baking sheet with cornmeal; set aside.

Prepare Italian Herb Filling. In a small bowl, mix mozzarella cheese and parmesan cheese. Punch down dough. Roll dough into a 16x12 inch rectangle. Place on prepared sheet. Place filling lengthwise down center third of dough. Sprinkle cheese mixture on top of filling. Make diagonal cuts 2 inches apart from edge of dough to filling. Crisscross diagonal strips over filling. Lightly spray top of loaf with water and sprinkle with sesame seeds. Bake in preheated oven 20–25 minutes or until golden brown.

Kid-Friendly Recipe: Reserve some of the bread dough, to form 4-inch circles of dough, rolled out to about ¼-inch thick. Top the bottom half of each dough round with cheese and a 2 Tbsp. meat mixture. Fold the top half of dough over the bottom to form a half circle. Pinch the sides down with the tines of a fork, and then prick several holes in the top of each pillow to allow steam to escape when baking. Brush with melted butter and a little parmesan cheese. Bake at 350 degrees until golden brown.

chicken florentine

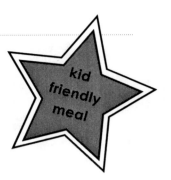

2 pkgs. frozen chopped spinach
¼ cup butter
1 garlic clove, crushed
dash basil and thyme
¼ cup flour
⅓ cup whipping cream
5 cups cooked chicken, sliced
¾ cups half and half
¾ cups chicken broth
salt and pepper to taste
6 thin slices ham
1 cup grated parmesan

Cook spinach according to package directions. Drain well. In a skillet, melt 1 tablespoon butter; add minced garlic, basil, and thyme. Cook over medium heat, stirring constantly for 5 minutes. Add 1 Tbsp. flour, and blend well. Add ⅓ cup whipping cream and spinach. Simmer 5 minutes. Put spinach into the bottom of a lightly buttered 2-quart baking dish. Cover with cooked chicken slices over medium low heat. Melt remaining butter and blend in remaining flour, stirring until smooth. Gradually stir in ¾ cup half-and-half and ¾ cup chicken broth. Continue cooking and stirring until thickened. Season with salt and pepper. Cut sliced ham in strips. Add to sauce and pour over chicken. Cover the whole lot with parmesan cheese, and bake at 400 degrees for 20 minutes or until cheese is lightly browned.

Kid-Friendly Recipe: Cook the bowtie pasta as recommended, and top with the white sauce as directed. Serve alongside a small salad of fresh spinach and sliced strawberries.

grilled lemon chicken
and Coconut Rice

½ cup lemon flavored yogurt
1 tsp. ground cumin
½ cup seasoned rice vinegar
¼ tsp. pumpkin pie spice
1-inch piece ginger, minced
1½ lbs. boneless chicken thighs or breasts
2 garlic cloves, minced
skewers (if wooden, soak in water 15 minutes)

Light charcoal briquettes or preheat broiler. In a large glass or plastic bowl, combine yogurt, rice vinegar, ginger, garlic, cumin, pie spice, ½ tsp. salt, and ¼ teaspoon pepper; set aside. Pound chicken to ½- inch thickness; cut into 1½-inch wide strips. Add chicken to yogurt mixture; toss to coat. Cover; refrigerate at least 20 minutes or up to 24 hours. Thread chicken onto skewers; spoon marinade over both sides of chicken. Discard any remaining marinade. Grill or broil chicken until no longer pink in the center, about 3-4 minutes per side. Serve with potato salad.

Coconut Rice

1 cup coconut milk
1 cup water
1 cup rice
2 Tbsp. butter

½ tsp. salt
1 cinnamon stick
⅛ tsp. ginger
orange zest

In a rice cooker or small saucepan, cook rice in coconut milk, water, butter, and salt. When rice is almost tender, add cinnamon stick, ginger, and orange zest. Simmer on low 4 minutes. When rice is tender, remove the cinnamon stick, and mix rice well. Serve alongside the chicken skewers.

ultimate shrimp scampi

1 (16-oz.) pkg. angel hair pasta
1 dash Worcestershire Sauce
½ cup butter
¼ cup lemon juice
4 cloves garlic, minced
1 lb. cooked shrimp
½ cup minced onion
½ cup Asiago cheese, diced
1 Tbsp. chopped fresh parsley
1 large avocado, peeled, pitted and diced
½ tsp. black pepper

Bring water to a boil, and cook pasta until al dente. Drain. Melt butter in a large skillet and stir in the garlic, onion, parsley, salt, pepper, Worcestershire sauce, and lemon juice. Once the mixture begins to bubble, increase the heat to medium-high, and stir in the shrimp. Cook and stir until the shrimp turn pink, and are no longer transparent in the center, about 5 minutes. Serve the scampi over a bed of angel hair pasta, and sprinkle with Asiago cheese and avocado to serve.

about the author

Anitra Kerr resides in Holladay, Utah. She is married and is the mother of four boys. As a professional organizer, personal coach, and master teacher, Anitra dedicates much of her time to teaching women how to find balance in their lives through organization, effective meal planning, home storage, and of course, personal time-out. As co-creator of the website www.simplylivingsmart.net, Anitra has been instrumental in teaching families worldwide how to use their personal resources to become more self-reliant and more confident in their ability to take care of the ones they love. She offers web-based training that focuses on concepts of food storage and meal planning as well as everyday organization in the home. She teaches weekly seminars and is also the author of, *Simply Living Smart—Everyday Solutions for a More Organized You*. Anitra's personal coaching has been one of her greatest loves. She works side by side with women in their homes, helping them to understand the value of living an organized, stress-free life.